Fracture Management

Field Guide *to* Fracture Management

RICHARD B. BIRRER, M.D., F.A.A.F.P., F.A.C.S.M.

Professor of Medicine
Cornell University Joan and Sanford I. Weill
Medical College and Graduate School of Medical Sciences
New York, New York
President and CEO
St. Joseph's Healthcare System
Paterson, New Jersey

ROBERT L. KALB, M.D.

Adjunct Professor
University of Toledo
Orthopedic Surgeon, Clinical Instructor
Bone, Joint, and Spine Surgeons
Toledo, Ohio

LIPPINCOTT WILLIAMS & WILKINS
A **Wolters Kluwer** Company
Philadelphia · Baltimore · New York · London
Buenos Aires · Hong Kong · Sydney · Tokyo

Acquisitions Editor: Danette Somers
Editorial Assistant: Mary Choi
Project Manager: Alicia Jackson
Senior Manufacturing Manager: Benjamin Rivera
Marketing Manager: Kathy Neely
Designer: Risa Clow
Production Service: Silverchair Science + Communications
Printer: R R Donnelley-Crawfordsville

© 2005 by LIPPINCOTT WILLIAMS & WILKINS
530 Walnut Street
Philadelphia, PA 19106 USA
LWW.com

Library of Congress Cataloging-in-Publication Data

Birrer, Richard B.
  Field guide to fracture management / Richard B. Birrer, Robert L. Kalb.
    p. ; cm.
  Includes bibliographical references and index.
  ISBN 0-7817-3536-X
  1.   Fractures. 2.   Primary care (Medicine) I. Kalb, Robert L. II. Title.
    [DNLM: 1. Fractures–therapy. WE 180 B619f 2005]
  RD101.B545 2005
  617.1'5–dc22
                                                                                            2004020117

Care has been taken to confirm the accuracy of the information presented and to describe generally accepted practices. However, the authors, editors, and publisher are not responsible for errors or omissions or for any consequences from application of the information in this book and make no warranty, expressed or implied, with respect to the currency, completeness, or accuracy of the contents of the publication. Application of this information in a particular situation remains the professional responsibility of the practitioner.

The authors, editors, and publisher have exerted every effort to ensure that drug selection and dosage set forth in this text are in accordance with current recommendations and practice at the time of publication. However, in view of ongoing research, changes in government regulations, and the constant flow of information relating to drug therapy and drug reactions, the reader is urged to check the package insert for each drug for any change in indications and dosage and for added warnings and precautions. This is particularly important when the recommended agent is a new or infrequently employed drug.

Some drugs and medical devices presented in this publication have Food and Drug Administration (FDA) clearance for limited use in restricted research settings. It is the responsibility of health care providers to ascertain the FDA status of each drug or device planned for use in their clinical practice.

10 9 8 7 6 5 4 3 2 1

To our patients and colleagues

CONTENTS

CONTRIBUTING AUTHORS

Richard B. Birrer, M.D., F.A.A.F.P., F.A.C.S.M.
Professor of Medicine
Cornell University Joan and Sanford I. Weill Medical College and Graduate School of Medical Sciences
New York, New York
President and CEO
St. Joseph's Healthcare System
Paterson, New Jersey

Garrick A. Cox, M.D.
Chief Orthopaedic Resident
Department of Orthopaedic Surgery
Seton Hall University
St. Joseph's University Medical Center
Paterson, New Jersey

Manish K. Gupta, M.D.
Chief Orthopaedic Resident
Department of Orthopaedics
Seton Hall University
St. Joseph's University Medical Center
Paterson, New Jersey

Robert L. Kalb, M.D.
Adjunct Professor

University of Toledo
Orthopedic Surgeon, Clinical Instructor
Bone, Joint, and Spine Surgeons
Toledo, Ohio

David V. Lopez, M.D.
Chief Resident
Department of Orthopaedics
Seton Hall University
St. Joseph's University Medical Center
Paterson, New Jersey

Arthur W. Pallotta, M.D.
Resident
Department of Orthopaedics
Seton Hall University
St. Joseph's University Medical Center
Paterson, New Jersey

Mark M. Pizzurro, M.D.
Resident
Department of Orthopaedic Surgery
Seton Hall University
St. Joseph's University Medical Center
Paterson, New Jersey

PREFACE

The musculoskeletal system is usually "tiger country" for the busy primary care physician. Fractures, in particular, can be challenging to diagnose and treat because there is little time spent on the subject in the basic and clinical sciences during medical school. Although time is allocated to orthopedics in some primary care residencies, continuing education courses and actual practice are the typical means by which a primary care physician becomes comfortable recognizing and managing common fractures. These may range from straightforward long-bone fractures in the industrial setting to the occult stress fractures seen in athletic and recreational activities. The ability to manage fractures resulting from athletic and occupational injuries is important because, as the "captain of the ship," the primary care physician is responsible for the treatment of soft tissue injuries, the rehabilitation process, and overall reintroduction back into the athletic and occupational world. This field guide was designed for the busy primary care physician. The epidemiology, mechanism of injury, presentation, imaging evaluation, diagnosis, and treatment plan are succinctly presented to optimize outcome and minimize the pitfalls inherent in fracture management. Read, enjoy, and prosper.

Richard B. Birrer, M.D., F.A.A.F.P., F.A.C.S.M.
Robert L. Kalb, M.D.

ACKNOWLEDGMENTS

The authors wish to thank the staff of Lippincott Williams & Wilkins, especially Danette Somers, Mary Choi, and Alicia Jackson. We are very grateful to the faculty and residents of the Department of Orthopaedics at St. Joseph's University Medical Center, Paterson, New Jersey.

Field Guide *to*
Fracture
Management

Chapter 1

INTRODUCTION TO OFFICE FRACTURE MANAGEMENT

Robert L. Kalb

Primary care physicians are able to treat a wide range of fractures in the office and obtain good clinical outcomes. Your level of training and knowledge indicates the complexity of the fractures that you can treat. This chapter discusses the elements of strong fracture management skills: education, training, case selection, and orthopedic consultations. As a quick reference, insurance codes and billing information for fracture treatments are presented.

EDUCATION AND TRAINING

Fracture management training can be done through course work and preceptorships. This handbook serves as an important tool for reference and can be used as a guide for fracture evaluation and treatment during residency and in practice. The author also can recommend additional courses and arrange preceptorships.

Courses

The National Procedures Institute in Midland, Michigan (www.npinstitute.com), offers fracture courses directed toward primary care. Jack Pfenninger, a family physician, founded the institute, which has an outstanding reputation for teaching procedure skills. Course work includes workshops on cast and splint applications, x-ray review, and decision making in fracture management.

Preceptorship

A preceptorship with an orthopedic surgeon is an excellent way to obtain training. You should decide beforehand how much time you can devote toward training and the complexity of fracture management that you want to learn. To arrange a preceptorship, contact Robert L. Kalb, MD, (419) 472-3791, 3900 Sunforest Ct, Suite 119, Toledo, OH 43623.

CASE SELECTION

You should master simple cases of fracture management before you progress to cases with higher degrees of difficulty. *Simple fractures* are extraarticular, nondisplaced, and nonangulated. *Complex fractures* extend into the joint (intraarticular) or are displaced and angulated, possibly requiring reduction.

Fracture management for children and adults differs greatly. Children's fractures will be presented separately in this handbook. Case presentations include treatment options and variations, frequency of office follow-up visits, and pitfalls in fracture management. Fracture characteristics are discussed, such as appearance and force involved with the trauma causing the fracture. For example, fractures associated with motor vehicle accidents have more soft tissue damage and a greater chance for complications, such as nerve or vessel injury and compartment syndrome, than those fractures that occur from a fall in standing position at ground level.

TABLE 1   Coding Information

International Classification of Diseases, Ninth Revision, Clinical Modification Code	Description
829.0	Fracture (abduction) (adduction) (avulsion) (compression) (angulated) (crush) (dislocation) (oblique) (displaced) (closed)[a]
824.8	Ankle (malleolus) (closed)
818.0	Arm (closed)
819.0	Arms, both (any bones) [with rib(s)] (with sternum) (closed)
829.0	Bone (closed)
825.0	Calcaneus (closed)
814.00	Carpal bone(s) (wrist) (closed)
810.00	Clavicle (closed)
813.41	Colles' (reversed) (closed)
821.00	Femur, femoral (closed)
823.81	Fibula (closed)
817.0	Hand, multiple bones of one hand (closed)
820.8	Hip (closed)
812.20	Humerus (closed)
827.0	Leg (closed)
828.0	Legs, both (any bones, closed)
824.8	Malleolus (closed)
815.00	Metacarpus, metacarpal [bones(s)], of one hand (closed)
825.25	Metatarsus, metatarsal [bones(s)], of one foot (closed)
813.03	Monteggia's (closed)
814.01	Navicular, carpal (wrist) (closed)
733.82	Nonunion
808.8	Pelvis, pelvic [bone(s)] (with visceral injury) (closed)
826.0	Phalanx, phalanges, of one foot (closed)
816.00	Phalanx, phalanges, of one hand (closed)
813.81	Radius (alone) (closed)
825.22	Scaphoid
811.00	Scapula (closed)
825.21	Talus (ankle bone) (closed)
825.29	Tarsus, tarsal bone(s) (with metatarsus) of one foot (closed)
816.00	Thumb [and finger(s)] of one hand (closed)
823.80	Tibia (closed)
826.0	Toe(s) of one foot (closed)
823.41	Torus
813.82	Ulna (alone) (closed)
805.8	Vertebra, vertebral (back) (body) (column) (neural arch) (pedicle) (spine) (spinous process) (transverse process) (closed)
814.00	Wrist (closed)

[a]*Closed* includes the following descriptions of fractures: comminuted, torus (buckle), linear, greenstick, impacted.

Primary care physicians cannot treat all types of fractures. Some fractures require referral to an orthopedic surgeon.

CONSULTATION

Consultation with an orthopedist is appropriate when you are concerned about any fracture management issue. You also should invite consultation if a patient requests an additional opinion.

Consultation is recommended for displaced intraarticular fractures, because most require reduction. If you are comfortable with reduction of fractures that are intraarticular and displaced, you can proceed. If the postreduction films show continued intraarticular displacement, it is appropriate to refer to an orthopedist.

Primary care physicians can perform fracture reductions for the distal radius. Fingertrap traction is used to reduce these fractures. This will be discussed in Chapter 16, Fractures of the Forearm and Distal Radius.

Other fractures that require consultation include those that are open through the skin and those that remain unacceptably angulated.

REIMBURSEMENT

A complete list of insurance codes and billing information for common fractures is presented in Table 1. Fracture management with or without surgery is appropriately charged as a global charge, which includes the usual customary and reasonable fee for fracture treatment and also the office follow-up visits for 3 months from the date of fracture. This global fee does not include cast changes, x-rays, splints, or injections. During an office follow-up visit in this 3-month interval, if a patient also has another problem (e.g., hypertension), it is appropriate to charge and receive payment for that problem in addition to the fracture follow-up.

Chapter 2

EQUIPMENT NEEDED

Robert L. Kalb

Different types of equipment are needed to treat fractures in the office. This chapter presents the equipment that is necessary for fracture management.

CAST EQUIPMENT

Cast Saw

You should become very familiar with operating a cast saw (Fig. 1) so that you do not burn or cut a patient's skin. The cast saw blade does not turn 360 degrees, as one would expect. Rather, it rotates back and forth in an arc of 30 degrees, which helps prevent cutting the skin.

The technique for operating a cast saw involves holding your hand against the saw with a finger from the hand bridging to the cast, so that if the patient moves the cast, the saw moves along with the cast. This technique is similar to that of using the otoscope on a child: One holds the otoscope with fingers making contact with the child's head, so that if the child moves his or her head, the otoscope moves as a unit rather than plunging into the ear canal. The proper technique for using a cast saw involves pushing the saw slowly downward through the cast material and then raising the saw completely from the cast and moving in a line toward the end of the cast. At each step of the way, the cast saw takes small 1-in. bites, vertically cutting the cast much as one would perforate paper. This is different from moving the cast saw in a line at the same depth, which can result in cutting the skin. If the cast saw blade becomes hot, turn off the cast saw and let it cool before continuing. This prevents the skin from burning.

There are a variety of saw models and costs. You should choose a cast saw that is affordable. The more expensive models have the advantage of being more quiet and less frightening for patients. If plaster is frequently used, it is wise to have a vacuum canister hooked to the cast saw to prevent dust in the room.

Cast Spreader

The cast spreader (Fig. 2A, B, and C) works in the opposite way of pliers. When the handle is pressed, the flat surfaces on the end of the cast spreader move in opposite directions, resulting in the cast splitting open along the saw cut line.

Cast Bender

The cast bender (Fig. 2D) is valuable for softening or turning out the margins of the cast where the cast can cut into skin or become sharp at the edges that contact skin. The cast bender is very similar to household pliers. You can grab the end of the cast and bend it outward, like pliers are used to shape the edge of a metal container.

LINER MATERIAL

Webril

The cast padding is made of cotton or synthetic material. The cotton Webril (Fig. 3) is easier to apply than the synthetic material. The synthetic Webril is

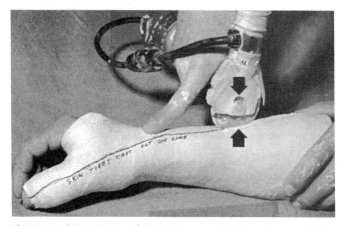

Figure 1   A felt marker is useful for writing on casts. When using an oscillating saw, be sure the blade is sharp and does not overheat. Use one finger as a fulcrum on the cast to stabilize the blade and cut by pushing downward (*down arrow*) and pulling upward (*up arrow*) when the cast saw is moved along. Avoid bony prominences. Never draw the saw longitudinally, as it can cut skin.

more expensive and is more difficult to tear during the application. The only advantage of synthetic Webril is that it tends to hold less moisture and therefore has an advantage in warm, humid climates in conjunction with the use of fiberglass cast materials. Cotton Webril can be used with fiberglass or plaster casting materials.

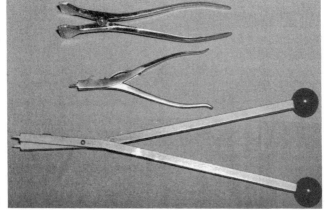

Figure 2   Cast spreaders. **A:** A two-handed cast spreader. **B:** Cast spreader designed to be used with one hand: The thin tine is quite useful. **C:** Another two-handed cast spreader that uses the same tine principle as **B**. (*continues*)

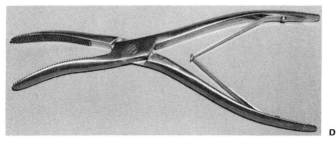

D

Figure 2 *Continued.* **D:** A cast bender for softening the edges of casts.

Gore-Tex Padding

Gore-Tex (Fig. 4) (W. E. Gore Co., Flagstaff, AZ) makes a cast padding material that can be used to make a waterproof swimming cast along with fiberglass cast material. This application is most appropriate for warm, moist climates and the summer season when people are swimming. Patients can even go scuba diving with a long-leg fiberglass cast and Gore-Tex padding without difficulty.

CASTING MATERIAL

Fiberglass

Fiberglass (Fig. 5) is a casting material that is less forgiving and more difficult to apply than plaster. If any pressure points occur with the fiberglass cast, they must be removed by making a cast window. Fiberglass has several advantages: It is lightweight and waterproof, and fractures are more visible when x-rays are taken through the fiberglass.

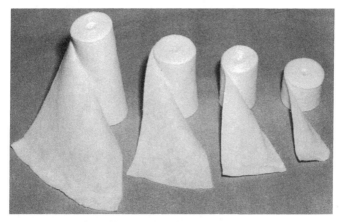

Figure 3 Webril for padding casts comes in rolls in widths of 2, 3, 4, and 6 in.

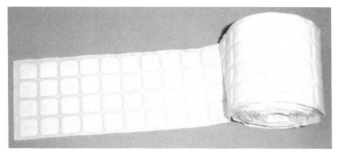

Figure 4   Gore-Tex.

Plaster Roll

Plaster (Fig. 6) is less expensive than fiberglass and has the advantages of a longer working time and a lower risk of pressure sores over prominent areas of bone, such as the distal ulna at the dorsal wrist.

SPLINT MATERIAL

Fiberglass

Splint material is identical to the fiberglass rolls. It is packaged in a watertight, airtight foil pouch. You can make fiberglass splints by taking a roll of fiberglass and rolling it out and back and forth on itself to form several layers in a

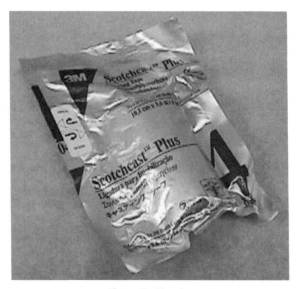

Figure 5   Fiberglass.

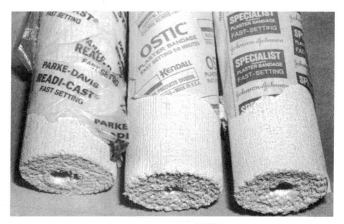

Figure 6   Plaster of Paris rolls are available in widths of 2, 3, 4, 5, 6, and 8 in.

straight line. Any air perforations or leaks in the airtight pouches allow the chemical reaction to begin, and the fiberglass will become hard. If a roll of fiberglass or a pack of fiberglass splint material is opened and has hard areas, it should be discarded. Your fiberglass supplier will usually replace this material free of charge.

Plaster Splints for Cast Reinforcement

Plaster splints (Fig. 7) are the same material as a roll of plaster rolled out to length and cut in various lengths and thicknesses. Plaster does not require an airtight container and is wrapped in wax paper. Plaster has a much longer shelf life than fiberglass.

Prepadded, One-Step, Stand-Alone Splints

The splint material comes in packages of various lengths and widths. This splint material is available with foam padding attached. This is ideal for easy office splint application, because it is prepadded. The foam attached to the fiberglass takes the place of the Webril padding. This prepadded splint material is also available in a plaster form. Prepadded plaster splints have no advantage over fiberglass, and the cost is the same. The prepadded fiberglass material on a roll has a resealable clasp mechanism. After opening, the package can be sealed to protect the remaining material. If this clasp should leak and air gets inside, the material usually hardens at the end, but the hard part can be cut off and discarded. Orthoglass is a prepadded fiberglass splint material in rolls of 2-, 3-, 4-, 5-, and 6-in. size. The 3- and 6-in. sizes are most commonly used. The 6-in. size is necessary for boxer fractures and also can be used for posterior leg splints. The 3-in. size is ideal for wrist, elbow, and long-arm splints.

ACCESSORIES

- Cast scissors (Fig. 8) are heavy-duty bandage scissors that require frequent sharpening and are designed to cut heavy cast padding, such as Webril, fiberglass, or plaster. They are not intended for cutting fiberglass and plaster after it has hardened.

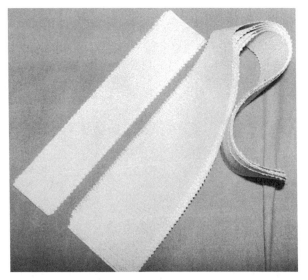

Figure 7 Plaster splints are available in many sizes. Use them in multiple layers to create adequate strength.

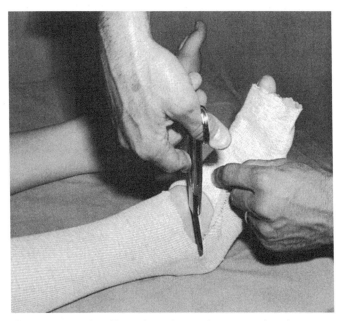

Figure 8 To avoid wrinkles in the stockinet under casts, cut along the concave surface of joints.

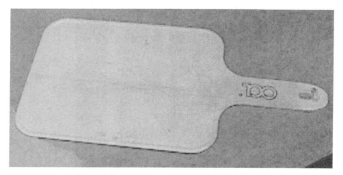

Figure 9 Cutting board for splint on a roll.

- Cutting board (wood or plastic) (Fig. 9). You should cut the fiberglass splint material with a heavy-duty linoleum knife on a board to protect your counter surface.
- Drop cloth. Material protects the floor and surface of the examination table from plaster and fiberglass.
- Gloves. Nonsterile gloves are mandatory when you are working with fiberglass and are recommended for working with plaster.
- Lubrication material. K-Y jelly or hand lotion can be used on the outer layers of the fiberglass cast to prevent layer separation.
- Ace wrap bandages. These bandages are useful for wrapping the cast while it is hardening when fiberglass is used. The Ace wrap bandage can be left in place to protect other skin areas from being scratched by the rough surface of the fiberglass. The wrap can be removed and washed if it becomes soiled and then reapplied to the cast for protection and padding.
- Cast boot (Fig. 10). A cast boot is important to protect the toes and keep the cast dry when patients are walking outdoors. It also prevents foreign

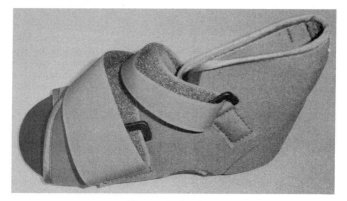

Figure 10 Cast boot.

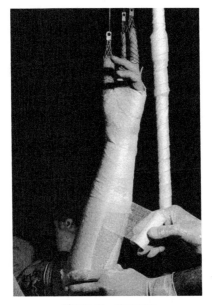

Figure 11 Fingertrap.

material from entering the end of the cast around the toes, resulting in puncture wounds, such as from a wood splinter or pin on the floor.
- Fingertrap (Fig. 11). Chinese fingertraps are the standard device for reducing distal radius fractures. (They work by the same principle as those found in toy shops or carnivals.) To protect the skin from the pull of the metal material in the fingertrap, apply adhesive tape over the finger to act as a layer of padding.
- Cast stand (Fig. 12). This device is extremely valuable for holding the patient's foot at a 90-degree angle during cast or splint application. The patient sits over the edge of the examination table and rests the foot on the adjustable-height foot stand. The bar supporting the foot is only 2 in. wide and $1/2$ in. in thickness. The bar attaches to the stand beyond the toes and has a blunt end that extends back to support the heel. The cast is applied to the foot with the ankle held in the neutral position so that the foot forms a 90-degree angle with the long axis of the tibia. This causes the heel cord to be under tension so that it does not become tight due to the cast being applied in a plantar-flexed, equinus position. After the cast hardens, the cast stand is pulled forward away from the toes. It is easily removed from the cast padding–skin interface.
- Goniometer (Fig. 13). A goniometer functions as a protractor to determine the angle measurement associated with fractures. It is held against an x-ray at the fracture site to measure the degree of angulation at the fracture site. A goniometer can be obtained from a cast supply vendor. Attach the goniometer to your x-ray view box along with a No. 1 lead pencil so that lines can be drawn on the x-ray and measured with the goniometer.

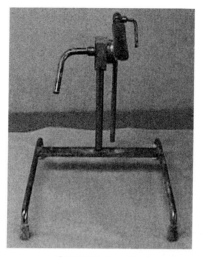

Figure 12 Cast stand.

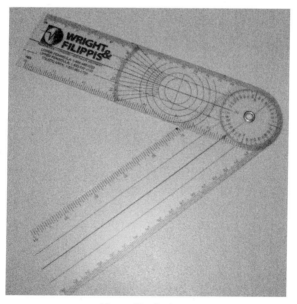

Figure 13 Goniometer.

Chapter 3

TERMS AND DEFINITIONS

Robert L. Kalb

This chapter presents the terms, definitions, and descriptions of fractures and fracture management.

DISPLACEMENT

The bone is separated at the fracture site, and there is an offset. Displacement can be measured in millimeters or centimeters, or as a percentage. A tibia fracture that is transverse with the distal end displaced by one-third of the cortex diameter has 33% posterior displacement (Fig. 1).

Displacement is always mentioned with reference to the bone end proximal to the fracture site. For example, a fracture of the tibial shaft where the distal fragment is sitting anterior by 50% of the cortical width would have 50% anterior displacement. Lateral, posterior, and medial displacement would also be described in this manner.

ANGULATION

Angulation of the fracture site refers to the angle made at the apex of the fracture site. For example, in a tibia fracture, if there is a 30-degree bend at the fracture site, it would be considered 30 degrees angulated (Fig. 2).

The angulation is described where the apex of the angle points. For example, a tibia fracture that is pointing medially would be described as having 30 degrees of medial angulation, or one could say that the apex of the angle points medially to describe the fracture. A fracture may have both angular deformity and displacement. A fracture could be angulated without displacement or be displaced without angulation.

CLOSED FRACTURES

The fracture is enclosed by soft tissue, and the overlying skin is intact. These are the most common fractures.

OPEN FRACTURES (PREVIOUSLY CALLED *COMPOUND FRACTURES*)

The bone breaks through the skin. There are three types of open fractures: *Type I* is characterized by an inside-out puncture from the sharp edge of the bone pushing through the skin, resulting in a laceration of less than 1 cm. Blood may leak through these lacerations. These fractures can be treated as closed injuries. The wound also can be washed in a sterile environment in the operating room.

A *type II fracture* has a laceration larger than 1 cm and is often associated with contamination at the fracture site from foreign material such as clothing or carpet fibers. These fractures always require irrigation and débridement in the operating room as an emergency.

A *type III fracture* is a wound larger than 5 cm and always requires emergency irrigation and débridement in the operating room. All open fracture

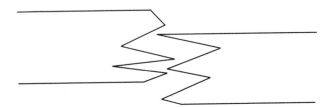

Figure 1   30% displacement, as the bone has displaced 30% of its diameter.

types I, II, or III should be referred because of the increased liability associated with the increased incidence of infection.

COMMINUTED FRACTURE

The comminuted fracture has more than two parts: It splinters into two main pieces and a third piece off one edge. This third piece is often referred to as a *butterfly fragment* because of its shape.

Comminuted fractures are caused by high traumatic force. They are associated with a higher incidence of nonunion as the amount of force causes devascularization of the bone. They are associated with more soft tissue damage, hematoma, compartment syndrome, and skin damage. These fractures are more complicated and can be referred to an orthopedic surgeon.

PATHOLOGIC FRACTURE

A pathologic fracture occurs when a bone breaks from a force that would not ordinarily cause a bone to fracture. Conditions such as osteoporosis, bone cyst, tumor, or infection at the fracture site predispose the bone to crack.

A pathologic fracture can be characterized by a unique fracture pattern described as resembling a ripe banana—it looks like a banana, broken into two equal parts. The crack is transverse and noncomminuted, much like breaking a piece of chalk into two pieces.

Fractures in healthy bone rarely occur in this manner. Tumors that are metastatic to bone include the ovary, testicle, breast, lung, and prostate. All metastatic bone lesions are lytic except for prostate. A prostate metastasis

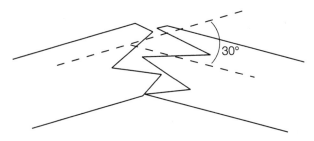

Figure 2   The angle subtended by the intersection of the lines in the illustration represents 30 degrees of angulation at the fracture site.

results in increased density, as it is a bone-forming tumor. The bone is weakened because the bone formation is not along lines of stress but rather is haphazard. Metastatic tumors to bone rarely, if ever, go below the elbow or the knee. If there is a lesion on the bone below the elbow or the knee, it is unlikely to be due to metastatic cancer.

If patients who are 50 years old or older report night pain, consider a tumor as the possible cause of the pain with metastasis to bone. Order a bone scan. If there is also concern about infection, a three-phase bone scan should be specified. Night pain is a red-flag, or danger signal, symptom.

Pathologic fractures also occur when a patient has disuse osteoporosis from bed rest or paralysis. When an individual becomes paralyzed, the non–weight-bearing femur and tibia do not work against the stress of gravity. As a result, the bone becomes weak, thin, and osteoporotic and is at high risk for fracture. It is common for a paralyzed patient to roll over in bed and break the femur. The bone is as thin as an eggshell. These fractures are treated with pillow splints and heal at the same rate as a normal bone. The healing rate of osteoporotic bone is not slower than that of healthy bone. Fracture union is always delayed by use of nicotine.

STRESS FRACTURES

Stress fractures occur when the bone is trying to remodel in response to stress. When repetitive loading stress is placed on a bone and the bone is not sufficiently strong to endure the stress, a rapid race between bone restoration/remodeling and tear-down occurs. If the repetitive loading stress continues, the tear-down portion of the remodeling job may occur at a more rapid rate than the new bone formation. This may result in bone pain and disuse. Disuse is a protective mechanism allowing the healing rate to progress without continued bone tear-down. The stress fracture can heal, and visible new bone formation can be seen on follow-up x-ray.

A bone scan is a good indicator of a stress fracture if the patient has had pain for 3 weeks or more. Magnetic resonance imaging is a more sensitive and specific indicator of a stress fracture. A stress fracture present in the femoral neck at the hip can be diagnosed immediately on magnetic resonance imaging, but the bone scan may take 3 days to show it.

REDUCTION

Reduction is the term used to describe setting a fracture or putting a dislocated joint back into position.

The straight line principle applies to all reductions. The shortest distance between two points is a straight line. If a toy railroad train derails, the easiest way to get all the rail cars back in line is to pull on the engine and the caboose. Similarly, when reducing a fracture or dislocation, applying traction in line with the limb results in the fracture fragments (or joint dislocation) with the attached muscles pulling everything into a straight line, thus causing the reduction.

Chapter 4

SPINE FRACTURES

Mark M. Pizzurro and Robert L. Kalb

Injuries of the spine may cause permanent neurologic deficit and may be life threatening. The spinal column is composed of several vertebrae spaced by cartilaginous discs, all supported by multiple ligaments. These elements surround and protect the spinal cord. The spine is divided into four anatomic areas: cervical, thoracic, lumbar, and sacrococcygeal. All vertebrae, except that of C-1, have a body, pedicles, lamina, facets, transverse processes, and a spinous process. Intervertebral discs are composed of an outer annulus fibrosis and an inner nucleus pulposus. The annulus provides support under tension, whereas the nucleus pulposus resists compression.

CERVICAL SPINE

The first two vertebrae of the spine, otherwise known as the *atlas* and *axis*, respectively, have different anatomy and function from the rest of the spine. Their anatomy allows for them to provide the majority of flexion and rotation of the cervical spine (C-spine). For these reasons, C-1 and C-2 are subject to unique stresses and injuries.

There is an increased risk of C-spine fractures in motor vehicle accidents (MVAs), diving injuries, or falls from heights. There is an increased risk of not diagnosing these fractures when patients are under the influence of drugs or alcohol or are unconscious.

Mechanism of Injury

The mechanism of injury can include flexion-extension, rotation, twisting, axial load, or compression forces. Flexion-extension injuries occur with MVAs and are very unstable. Axial loads result from a weight falling onto the head or from diving into shallow water, causing the body's weight to be driven onto the head and neck.

Diagnosis

The first consideration in diagnosis is the mechanism of injury. In the presence of a flexion-extension or axial-loading injury, there must be a suspicion of a C-spine injury. On physical examination, there may be tenderness over the soft tissues around the neck or over the spinous processes. Swelling or ecchymoses around the neck may be indicative of significant trauma. Head trauma, bruising, and lacerations may suggest force transferred to the neck. Loss of consciousness masks pain and neurologic deficits.

Radiology

If any possibility of C-spine injury is present, C-spine radiographs should be taken immediately, including open-mouth odontoid view, anteroposterior (AP) and lateral views (showing all seven cervical vertebrae), and oblique views of the C-spine. If there is any question of C-spine subluxation, dislocation, or fracture, a computed tomography scan should be obtained. In obese or muscular patients, the lower cervical vertebra may not be visible on the standard lateral radiograph. This visualization can be improved by taking a swimmer view or a shoulder pull-down view. The examiner stands at the foot of the bed and pulls down on both hands, preventing the shoulders from obscuring the spine.

The lateral view of the C-spine is the single most important view. The soft tissues should be examined, looking for displacement or widening of the soft tissue window anterior to the spine and behind the trachea. The alignment of the spinal column anterior and posterior to the vertebral body and spinous processes should be continuous. Any disruption may represent a fracture, subluxation, or dislocation. This view also shows fractures of the spinous processes. The open-mouth view allows for visualization of C-2 with the odontoid process and the alignment of the articulation of C-1 with C-2. Any obvious or questionable abnormality requires a computed tomography scan.

Initial Treatment

All patients with a C-spine injury should have a hard collar, and spine board imaging can be completed. Precautions include logrolling. Management begins with the ABCs of trauma. A complete neurologic examination must be performed, including extremity reflexes and a rectal examination.

Definitive Treatment

Once a patient is stabilized and all C-spine radiographs have been obtained, it may be necessary to perform an MRI or flexion-extension radiographs to further diagnose the injury.

Spinous process fractures represent a low-energy injury diagnosed by posterior tenderness. These so-called clay shoveler's fractures are seen on the lateral C-spine radiograph. These are avulsion fractures that result from a forceful flexion and extension. Historically, Georgia prisoners building roads injured their necks when the red clay would cling to the shovel, resulting in a sudden flexion-extension of the C-spine. These are stable injuries and are treated symptomatically with a soft collar and analgesics.

All other cervical injuries require consultation.

When to Refer

Any C-spine injury with loss of consciousness, neurologic impairment, or malalignment of the spinal column should be referred.

THORACIC SPINE

The thoracic spine is composed of 12 vertebrae. There are 12 ribs, which articulate with the spine at the transverse process. The presence of the rib cage makes the thoracic spine more rigid than the cervical and lumbar spines. Spinal cord injuries at this level can result in paraplegia and difficulty with respiration, as the intercostal muscles may be affected. The most common injury is compression.

Mechanism of Injury

Similar to the C-spine, there may be flexion-extension, rotation and twisting, or axial-loading injuries. These may result from falls from a height, diving accidents, MVAs, or jumping injuries. Flexion-distraction injuries can occur from the pull of a seat belt in an MVA. Most occur in elderly osteoporotic patients with minor flexion injury.

Diagnosis

There should be a suspicion of an injury to the spinal column based on the mechanism of injury. The patient may complain of mid-back pain. Tenderness and ecchymoses may be present over the spine. Exquisite tenderness over the spinous process may represent a flexion-distraction injury with posterior ligamentous disruption. With thoracic spine injuries, the intercostal nerves traveling beneath each rib may be damaged, causing radicular pain. In high-energy mechanisms such as MVAs and falls from a height, there is an association with lower-extremity fractures and dislocations, so the feet and ankles must be carefully examined.

Radiology

The AP and lateral thoracic spine radiographs can show spinous process fractures, compression fractures of the vertebral bodies, and associated rib fractures. When a thoracic injury is diagnosed or suspected, additional imaging of the remainder of the spine should also be obtained to rule out other injuries.

Initial Treatment

Initial treatment involves immobilization with a spine board and neurologic examination.

Definitive Treatment

Axial loading of the thoracic spine may result in a compression fracture and kyphosis. A *gibbus deformity* is an acute angulation of the thoracic spine at the level of the compression fracture. Each compression fracture in the thoracic spine diminishes the pulmonary function capacity by at least 3%. It is quite significant in elderly, osteoporotic smokers with chronic obstructive pulmonary disease who are predisposed to multiple compression fractures. The loss of vertebral height and degree of angulation are used to determine whether bracing, operative stabilization, or kyphoplasty is necessary. A brace is custom fitted and uses three-point fixation to stabilize the spine. It must be worn for 6 weeks whenever the patient is out of bed.

Multiple compression fractures may indicate plasmacytoma or multiple myeloma (plasmacytoma in multiple locations) associated with serum glutamic-oxaloacetic transaminase elevation, elevated sedimentation rate, and anemia. Serum and urine immunoelectrophoresis is also used to diagnose myeloma.

In selected cases, compression fractures may be treated with a kyphoplasty. This procedure, which may be done under local anesthesia with sedation, involves using a balloon to elevate the vertebral endplates, restoring alignment, and then injecting cement into the vertebral body to maintain the position. The cement is inserted under fluoroscopic imaging to ensure that there is no flow outside of the vertebrae and into the spinal cord. The stability of the fracture, as well as the extent of deformity, is used to determine the definitive treatment. In stable, less severe injuries, a thoracolumbosacral orthosis may be used (Fig. 1).

When to Refer

Patients with multiple compression fractures or a single compression fracture with greater than 50% loss of height or with intractable pain should be referred.

LUMBAR SPINE

The five vertebrae of the lumbar spine are the largest. Two injuries that are usually related to repetitive trauma are spondylolisthesis and spondylolysis.

Mechanism of Injury

The mechanisms of injury are flexion-extension and twisting injuries resulting from MVAs and high-energy trauma. A fall from a height or diving accident may result in an axial load, causing a compression or burst fracture.

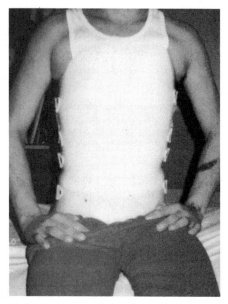

Figure 1   Anterior view of a patient fit with a custom thoracolumbosacral orthosis fabricated from a body cast mold. Note the contouring over the iliac crests.

Diagnosis

On examination, there may be tenderness and ecchymoses over the spinous processes. Neurologic deficit involving only the lower extremities may indicate a lumbar injury. A seat belt type of abrasion or ecchymoses may be present over the abdomen. Have a high suspicion in an unconscious patient and maintain immobilization precautions pending x-ray.

Radiology

The standard AP and lateral radiographs can show pathology in the lumbar spine. On the AP view, loss of a single pedicle, known as a *winking owl sign*, may indicate cortical destruction from a metastatic process. Fractures of the transverse processes can also easily be seen on this view. The lateral view allows visualization of compression and burst fractures as well as dislocations. Spondylolisthesis is the slipping of one vertebra on another. This can be diagnosed on the lateral view.

Fracture of the Pars Interarticularis

Spondylolysis is a term used to describe a fracture of the pars interarticularis. The pars interarticularis is the portion of the vertebra that connects the facet to posterior elements. These areas are commonly associated with lysis caused by stress fractures in the teenage years. They can be diagnosed on a routine lumbar spine film for back pain and are best seen on the oblique projections. They are almost never caused by sudden, violent trauma. Rather, they are stress fractures that occur over time, related to repeated hyperextension of the lumbar spine. This repeated hyperextension is common in football linemen and gymnasts. Repeated stress can result in a stress fracture and lysis at the L-5 vertebra pars interarticularis. If the lytic areas appear on a plain radiograph, the chance of healing is gone.

Appropriate treatment involves obesity prevention, no smoking, aerobic conditioning exercise, walking, bicycling, or swimming, and antiinflammatory medication. Surgical fusion is a last resort and is only indicated if the back pain remains intolerable and refractory to conservative treatment measures. A lumbar support can be used at work with instructions to avoid frequent bending, stooping, twisting, or lifting of more than 20 lb. Adults with an incidental finding of spondylolysis, with or without spondylolisthesis, do not have a higher incidence of back pain than the normal population without spondylolysis. These patients can pursue potentially physically demanding careers, such as firefighting or police work, or do physical labor without restriction provided that they are not symptomatic.

Initial Treatment

As with the thoracic spine, lumbar spine injuries should be immobilized with a spine board. Logrolling should be used in moving the patient. A complete neurologic and rectal examination must be done. In axial compression injuries with falls, the feet should be carefully examined to check for calcaneus fractures and tarsometatarsal injuries.

In the lumbar spine, the lumbar curvature is associated with normal lumbar lordosis. When one bends forward, the lordosis disappears and becomes a convex curvature rather than the lordotic concave curvature. If muscle spasm is present, when one bends forward, the normal lumbar lordosis does not reverse and become a convexity or kyphosis. This failure to reverse the normal lumbar lordosis is the only objective evidence of muscle spasm and should be documented in the chart. If this is not present, muscle spasm is not a proper diagnosis.

Burst fracture injuries are associated with axial-loading injuries such as parachute jumps or MVAs. These injuries are very unstable and can be associated with retropulsion of fragments from the vertebral body into the spinal canal.

Definitive Treatment

Correction may require surgery or brace immobilization. Braces that can be used for lumbar fracture stabilization as well as thoracic fracture stabilization cover the thoracic, lumbar, and sacral spines using three-point fixation as described for thoracic spine fractures.

When to Refer

Lumbar spine fractures with neurologic deficits should be referred to a specialist.

SACRAL FRACTURES

Sacral fractures most commonly occur with injuries to the pelvic ring. These are usually the result of high-energy trauma. Neurologic deficits involving the bladder and sphincter may be present.

Most isolated sacral fractures are stable and can be treated with bed rest followed by gradual mobilization with no weight bearing on the affected side. Fractures that occur with other pelvic injuries are discussed in Chapter 5. All sacral fractures with displacement or neurologic injury should be referred.

COMPLICATIONS

Any patient with paralysis or being treated with immobilization is at high risk for deep venous thrombosis, so placement of an inferior vena cava filter should be considered.

PELVIC FRACTURES

Mark M. Pizzurro and Robert L. Kalb

Fractures of the pelvis encompass a wide spectrum of injuries ranging from the simple pubic ramus fracture to the life-threatening open pelvis. Low-energy trauma usually results in pubic ramus injuries, which are treated symptomatically. In contrast, high-energy injuries, which occur most commonly from motor vehicle accidents, can include open fractures of the pelvis, acetabulum fractures with hip dislocations, and unstable pelvic ring fractures.

The pelvis consists of the sacrum and two innominate bones. The ischium, ilium, and pubis fuse at the triradiate cartilage to form the innominate bone (Fig. 1). The anterior ring is composed of the pubic and ischial rami, which meet at the pubic symphysis. During standing, weight is distributed from the sacrum to the iliac wing, acetabulum, and ischium, but not to the pubic rami (Fig. 2). Posteriorly, the innominate bones attach to the sacrum at the very strong sacroiliac joints.

One type of injury is the *avulsion fracture*, which occurs in skeletally immature patients at the site of a secondary ossification center where there is a muscular attachment, known as an *apophysis*. The apophysis is a growth plate that does not contribute to skeletal height. Figure 3 shows the many muscle attachments over the pelvis. Avulsions result from a single strong contraction or repetitive trauma during physical activity. Avulsion fractures can occur about the pelvis in adolescents over the anterior superior iliac spine from the pull of the sartorius muscle. A similar, but less common, avulsion fracture can occur at the anterior inferior iliac spine due to pull from the rectus femoris. Athletes who jump hurdles or gymnasts who do splits can avulse the ischial tuberosity. This area unites to the pelvis as late as at 25 years of age and, for that reason, can result in an avulsion fracture after adolescence.

Acetabular fractures, a separate category of pelvic fractures, result from high-energy trauma and often have associated injuries. Unlike the other pelvic ring injuries, acetabular fractures are intraarticular and must be reduced to as near an anatomic position as possible. Furthermore, there may be an associated hip fracture or dislocation, which is an emergency as there is a risk of avascular necrosis of the femoral head if not reduced in a timely fashion.

MECHANISM OF INJURY

Pelvis fractures can occur secondary to low- or high-energy injury. Low-energy injuries are fractures of the superior and inferior rami. These result from falls against a table or the floor in an osteoporotic patient, or from a height in a younger patient. Avulsion injuries occur during physical activity in which there is a strong contraction that pulls a muscle from its attachment on the pelvis.

The mechanism of a high-energy pelvis injury is a motor vehicle accident in most cases. Other common causes are pedestrian trauma, motorcycle accidents, and falls from heights. Life-threatening injuries such as hemorrhage,

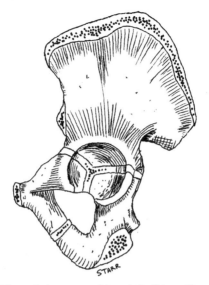

Figure 1   Immature pelvis and triradiate cartilage.

urethral or bladder disruption, and bowel perforation may accompany high-energy pelvis fractures.

DIAGNOSIS

A pelvis fracture should be suspected in any patient involved in a motor vehicle accident, pedestrian accident, or fall who complains of pelvic pain or is hemodynamically unstable. Such patients may have blood at the urethral meatus, open wounds over the pelvis, or ecchymoses around the pelvis and perineum. There may be hip or groin pain reproduced with movement of the lower extremity. Palpation and compression of the pelvis can elicit pain in the presence of any pelvic ring injury. In patients with a history of a low-energy fall, there may be difficulty bearing weight or walking or standing in conjunction with pain reproduced by palpation of the pelvis or gentle movement of the lower extremity. Injuries to the sacrum and sacroiliac joints cause local pain that is aggravated by direct palpation. Hip fractures and dislocations produce groin pain that is increased by rotation of the leg.

RADIOLOGY

The anteroposterior pelvis radiograph is part of all trauma evaluations. This film must be carefully reviewed, as some fractures can be obscured by an overlying object, such as a spine board. When there is a pelvic ring injury, inlet (40 degrees caudal) and outlet (40 degrees cephalad) views should be obtained (Figs. 4 and 5). If there is an acetabular fracture, the injury should be visualized with Judet views, otherwise known as *iliac* and *obturator obliques* (Figs. 6, 7, 8, and 9). These views allow for visualization of the anterior and posterior walls of the acetabulum as well as the supporting anterior and posterior columns of the pelvis.

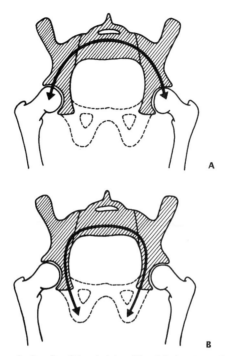

Figure 2   Standing **(A)** and sitting **(B)** weight-bearing arches.

INITIAL TREATMENT

In patients who are hemodynamically stable, a complete evaluation should be performed, including appropriate radiographs and computed tomography scans. Initial hemoglobin levels should be checked and followed at regular intervals for 24 hours or until stabilized. Isolated pubic ramus fractures are stable injuries, so these patients can walk, weight bearing as tolerated. Many of these patients require hospital admission for analgesics and physical therapy. Avulsion fractures are managed with bed rest, ice, and analgesics.

High-energy injuries require a complete trauma evaluation. Because of the association with other injuries, the entire skeleton must be examined. Management begins with the ABCs of trauma. Resuscitation and fluid replacement are the first two priorities. A pelvic binder or external fixator may be applied to stabilize a hemodynamically unstable patient with an open-book pelvic injury with resultant hemorrhage (Fig. 10).

DEFINITIVE TREATMENT

Low-energy injuries, including pubic and ischial ramus fractures as well as avulsion fractures, are treated symptomatically. Elderly patients are treated with analgesics and physical therapy. Typically, it may take a few days for them to return to ambulatory status. Progression to weight bearing is done gradually over the first few weeks. Avulsion fractures of the apophysis of the ante-

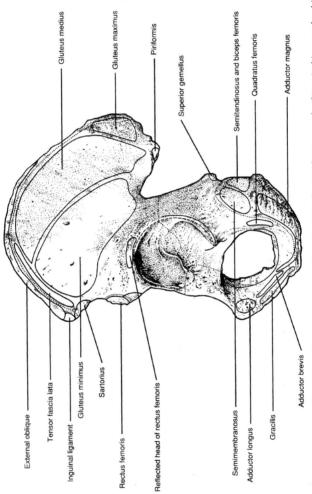

Figure 3 Lateral projection of the left innominate bone. Note the muscular attachments to the ilium, ischium, and pubis.

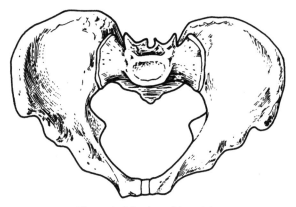

Figure 4   Inlet view of the pelvis.

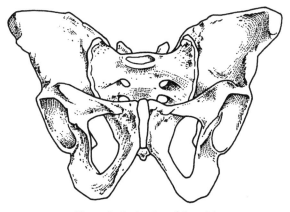

Figure 5   Outlet view of the pelvis.

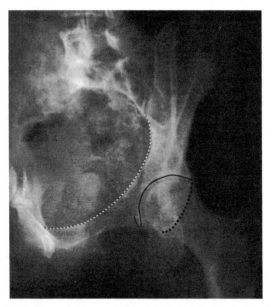

Figure 6 Obturator oblique x-ray of the left hemipelvis. This view is taken by elevating the affected hip 45 degrees to the horizontal by means of a wedge and directing the beam through the hip joint with a 15-degree upward tilt.

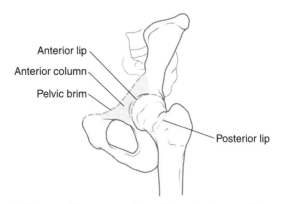

Figure 7 Diagram of the anatomy of the pelvis on the obturator oblique view. In this view, note particularly the pelvic brim, indicating the border of the anterior column and the posterior lip of the acetabulum. (From Tile M. *Fractures of the pelvis and acetabulum*. Baltimore: Williams & Wilkins, 1984, with permission.)

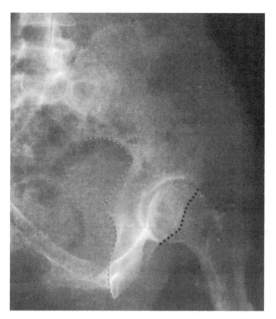

Figure 8 Iliac oblique radiographic view of the left hemipelvis. This view is taken by rotating the patient into 45 degrees of external rotation by elevating the uninjured side on a wedge.

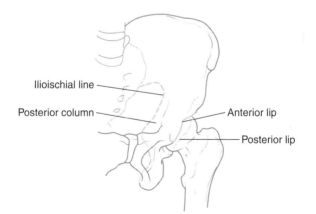

Figure 9 Diagram of the anatomic landmarks of the left hemipelvis on the iliac oblique view. This view best demonstrates the posterior column of the acetabulum, outlined by the ilioischial line, the iliac crest, and the anterior lip of the acetabulum. (From Tile M. *Fractures of the pelvis and acetabulum*, 2nd ed. Baltimore: Williams & Wilkins, 1995, with permission.)

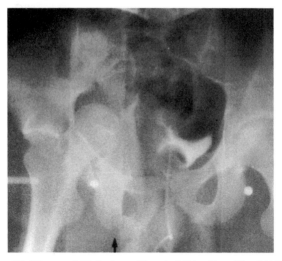

Figure 10   T-type unstable fracture with central dislocation of the right hip in a 23-year-old man. Note the displacement of the bladder to the left side and the fracture through the inferior ramus of the right pubis, which helps to delineate the T-type nature of this fracture (*arrow*). A general anesthetic was required to reduce the hip from within the pelvis.

rior superior and inferior iliac spines can be treated with flexion and abduction of the hip. Patients with ischial tuberosity avulsions are more comfortable with leg extension and external rotation.

WHEN TO REFER

Nearly all pelvis fractures require orthopedic consultation. All high-energy injuries require immediate orthopedic evaluation. Hip dislocation is an emergency and must be treated within a few hours of the injury due to the high risk for avascular necrosis of the femoral head.

COMPLICATIONS

There are several serious complications with pelvic and acetabular fractures. Thromboembolism is a major risk due to the disruption of the pelvic vasculature and immobilization required for treatment. Sequential compression devices for the legs should be used. Chemoprophylaxis and inferior vena cava filter placement may be used. Internal bleeding must be considered before the use of anticoagulants. Infection is also a major complication. This can occur secondary to ruptured bowel, in which case the mortality rate is 50%. Malunion of pelvic and acetabular fractures can result in chronic pain, leg length inequality, gait abnormalities, difficulties sitting, and pelvic outlet obstruction. With acetabular fractures, there is a significant risk of avascular necrosis of the femoral head. Posttraumatic arthritis is always a risk with intraarticular fractures.

Chapter 6

FEMORAL FRACTURES

Manish K. Gupta and Robert L. Kalb

FEMORAL NECK FRACTURE

Femoral neck fractures are the second most common hip fracture of the 280,000 that occur each year. These occur in two populations. Five percent are in young adults with high-energy injuries, whereas 95% are in elderly with underlying osteoporosis.

Mechanism of Injury

In the elderly, femoral neck fractures result from a fall while standing. Three common mechanisms are
1. Fall directly onto the greater trochanter
2. Lateral rotation with sudden increase in load
3. Spontaneous completion of a stress fracture that causes the fall (incidence increased with severity of osteoporosis)

Diagnosis

The patient may present with a history of hip pain over weeks and then a sudden fall due to a stress fracture. Pain with walking occurs in a nondisplaced fracture. There is inability to walk with displaced fractures. On physical examination, note shortening and rotation of the leg and pain with palpation of the hip and with range of motion.

Radiology

Anteroposterior (AP)/lateral views should be used to evaluate the fracture line and to assess degenerative arthritis. If no fracture line is seen and index of suspicion is high for fracture, get a magnetic resonance imaging scan (Fig. 1).

Initial Treatment

Bed rest with Buck's traction, 5 lb on affected extremity, to prevent motion. Prevent blood clots by placing calf pumps and start enoxaparin (Lovenox) low-molecular-weight heparin. Make sure to discontinue Lovenox 12 hours preoperatively. A medical consultation is needed for surgical clearance. Draw preoperative laboratory tests: prothrombin time/partial thromboplastin time, complete blood cell count, chemistry profile, electrocardiogram, chest x-ray, and urinalysis. Do all in emergency room on admission to avoid delay in medical clearance.

Definitive Treatment

For all fractures, orthopedic evaluation is warranted. Nondisplaced fractures can be treated with non–weight bearing for 6 to 8 weeks; however, surgical treatment is best if pain is severe. For displaced fractures, surgical treatment with prosthetic replacement (hemiarthroplasty) is standard. Deep venous thrombosis (DVT) prophylaxis is continued 4 weeks postoperatively with fondaparinux (Arixtra), 2.5 mg q.d. Rehabilitation goals are to decrease pain and resume walking to prevent complications of sepsis, skin ulcers, pneumonia, bowel dysfunction, and DVT.

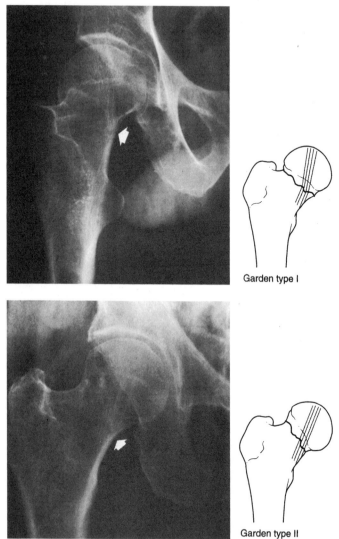

A

Garden type I

B

Garden type II

Figure 1 The Garden classification of femoral neck fractures. Type I fractures can be incomplete, but much more typically, they are impacted into valgus and retroversion **(A)**. Type II fractures are complete but undisplaced. These rare fractures have a break in the trabeculations, but no shift in alignment **(B)**. Type III fractures have marked angulation but usually minimal to no proximal translation of the shaft **(C)**. In the Garden type IV fracture, there is complete displacement between fragments, and the shaft translates proximally **(D)**. The head is free to realign itself within the acetabulum, and the primary compressive trabeculae of the head and acetabulum realign (*white lines*).

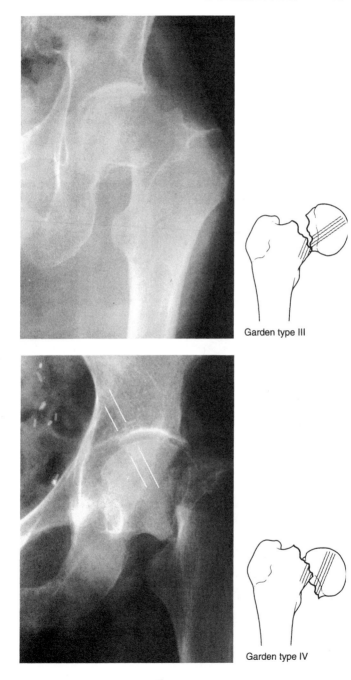

Garden type III

C

Garden type IV

D

FEMORAL INTERTROCHANTERIC FRACTURE

Femoral intertrochanteric fracture is the most common hip fracture in the elderly. This fracture is extracapsular and involves the greater and lesser trochanteric areas of the hip. Its incidence increases with age. It is more common in women than in men due to osteoporosis.

Mechanism of Injury

Injury results from a fall on the greater trochanter. In young patients, a femoral intertrochanteric fracture is rare and related to high-energy injuries such as motor vehicle accidents and falls from a height.

Diagnosis

Suspect a femoral intertrochanteric fracture in patients with a history of a fall and inability to walk. Physical examination shows shortened and externally rotated leg. There is pain on palpation of the hip and with range of motion of the hip.

Radiology

AP/lateral views of hip show the fracture line through the greater and lesser trochanter (Fig. 2).

Initial Treatment

Initial treatment should include surgical consultation with an orthopedist; bed rest with Buck's traction of 5 lb on affected extremity; preoperative laboratory

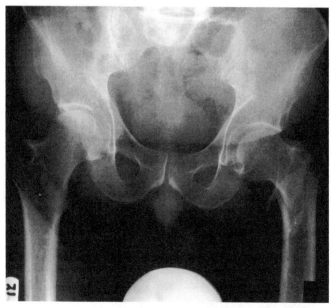

A

Figure 2 Anteroposterior view of the pelvis **(A)** and an anteroposterior **(B)** and a cross-table lateral **(C)** view of the hip showing a left intertrochanteric fracture.

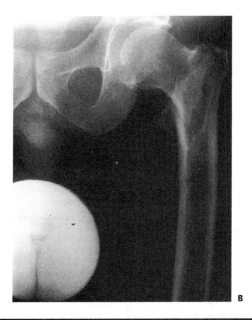

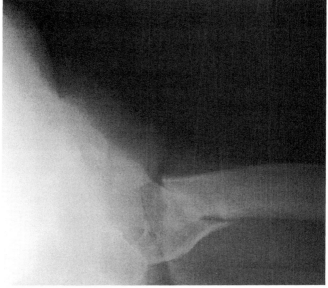

tests and medical consultation to clear for surgery; calf pumps and Lovenox for preoperative DVT prophylaxis; and Arixtra postoperatively for 1 month.

Definitive Treatment

Definitive treatment consists of reduction of the fracture and stabilization with compression plate and hip screw to achieve union. The rehabilitation goal is to walk to decrease complications of mortality, sepsis, and DVT.

FEMORAL SUBTROCHANTERIC AND SHAFT FRACTURE

Femoral subtrochanteric and shaft fractures result from high-energy injuries associated with motor vehicle, pedestrian-versus-vehicle, motorcycle, and industrial accidents. These fractures require the immediate attention of an orthopedic surgeon and are often associated with other fractures. Subtrochanteric and shaft fractures can be associated with low-energy injury in the setting of osteoporosis or pathologic conditions in the proximal femur.

Mechanism of Injury

The mechanism of injury is a direct blow or indirect forces (i.e., a fall).

Diagnosis

Patient presents with pain and inability to weight bear on the extremity. Fracture deformity, shortening, and rotational malalignment are obvious in the leg on physical examination.

Radiology

AP/lateral views of the proximal hip, pelvis, and shaft are necessary. Fracture lines extend from below the lesser trochanter and shaft.

Initial Treatment

Orthopedic surgical consultation is a must. Temporary splinting with traction en route to surgery is warranted. All preoperative laboratory tests are drawn in the emergency room to clear the patient for surgery.

Definitive Treatment

Surgical stabilization with an intramedullary rod is the treatment of choice. Rehabilitation goals are to gain union of the fracture, walk, and return to previous level of function. Complications can include infection, nonunion, malunion, implant failure, and DVT.

FRACTURES OF THE DISTAL FEMUR

Distal femur fractures are less common than hip fractures. They involve the distal 15 cm of the femur and can result in complications of angular deformity, joint incongruity, and knee stiffness.

Mechanism of Injury

These fractures are a result of severe varus, valgus, or rotational force with axial loading. These injuries are usually encountered in high-energy trauma, such as motor vehicle accidents and falls from heights.

Radiology

AP/lateral views of femur and knee are necessary. Displacement in the joint requires surgery (Fig. 3).

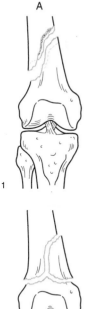
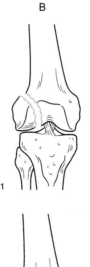
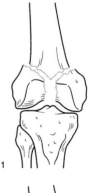
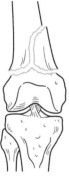
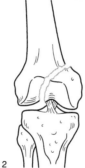
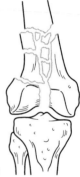
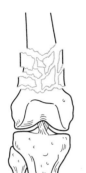
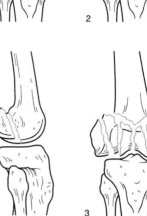

Figure 3 Orthopaedic Trauma Association classification of distal femur fractures. (Adapted from Orthopaedic Trauma Association Committee for Coding and Classification. Fracture and dislocation compendium. *J Orthop Trauma* 1996;10[Suppl 1]:41–45.)

Diagnosis

Patient presents with pain, swelling, and decreased range of knee motion. Physical examination shows deformity. If there is any vascular compromise or dislocation of the knee, obtain arteriography to examine the popliteal artery. Also obtain orthopedic consultation and order preoperative laboratory tests for surgery.

Initial Treatment

The affected extremity is splinted and placed in traction if surgery is delayed. If an open injury is present, the wound is irrigated in surgery and prophylactic antibiotics are started.

Definitive Treatment

If the fracture is undisplaced and the patient is too sick for surgery, this can be treated in a long-leg cast. Displaced fractures are reduced and stabilized internally with plates or rods. It is essential to restore joint line congruity to prevent complications of arthritis, stiffness, and deformity.

WHEN TO REFER

All femoral fractures benefit from an orthopedic evaluation, as most need operative treatment.

COMPLICATIONS

Most of the complications are nonunion, malunion, infection, DVT, and pulmonary embolus.

Chapter 7

PATELLAR FRACTURES

Manish K. Gupta and Robert L. Kalb

Patellar fractures account for 1% of all fractures and are usually seen in patients of ages 20 to 50 years. The patella is the largest sesamoid bone in the body and functions as a pulley to increase the power of the quadriceps tendon to extend the knee. Anatomically, it sits between the femoral condyles and is the attachment site for the quadriceps tendon superiorly and the patella tendon inferiorly.

MECHANISM OF INJURY

The majority of fractures occur from direct injuries to the patella, such as a fall or direct blow from an object. Dashboard injuries in motor vehicle accidents are also common. Indirect injuries can also occur, and these are usually secondary to soft tissue injuries resulting from twisting or jumping. An example is avulsion fracture secondary to pull of the quadriceps or patella tendon.

DIAGNOSIS

Pain, loss of motion, and inability to weight bear are the most common symptoms. Major signs are abrasion, swelling, or crepitus with inability to fully extend the knee from a flexed position (suggesting damage to the quadriceps or patella tendon). All lacerations should be checked to see if they communicate with the joint. (This can be checked by injecting saline in the joint to see if it extravasates from the wound.) If the test is positive, the knee joint requires surgical débridement as an emergency. If the knee x-ray shows air in the joint, the laceration goes into the knee.

RADIOLOGY

Anteroposterior/lateral, sunrise, and tunnel views are used. Lateral views in 30 degrees flexion are used to assess patella baja or alta (indicative of quadriceps tendon or patella tendon injury, respectively) and to evaluate fracture displacement. These views show if the patella is dislocated or subluxed (Fig. 1). Do not confuse an anatomic variant, bipartite patella, with a fracture (Fig. 2). This patella is nontender. It is always in the upper outer quadrant.

INITIAL TREATMENT

Pain control and immobilization are a priority. Doing a sterile arthrocentesis to evacuate blood from the knee joint relieves pain and improves motion. All cuts and abrasions should be cleaned and dressed. If the injury is closed, a knee immobilizer is applied and the patient can be discharged. If not, an orthopedic consultation is warranted.

DEFINITIVE TREATMENT

Closed fractures of the patella with separation less than 3 mm in the anteroposterior/lateral planes on radiographs, articular incongruity of less than 2

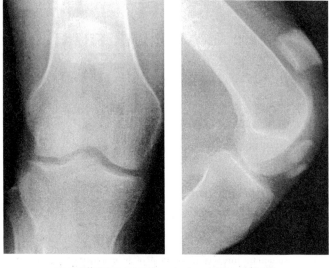

A,B

C

Figure 1 Anteroposterior **(A)**, lateral **(B)**, and sunrise **(C)** views of a displaced transverse patellar fracture.

mm, and intact quadriceps and patella tendons are treated with a knee immobilizer for 6 weeks. Patients may remove the knee immobilizer for a shower but must keep the knee straight. Maintain toe-touch weight bearing for 2 weeks and progress to full weight as the fracture heals. Follow up in 2 weeks after the initial visit with x-rays and then every 3 weeks until the fracture heals. The knee immobilizer is removed after 6 weeks when radiographic healing is present. Range of motion exercises and a quadriceps-strengthening program start at 6 weeks. Patients are fully recovered when quadriceps strength matches the unaffected side.

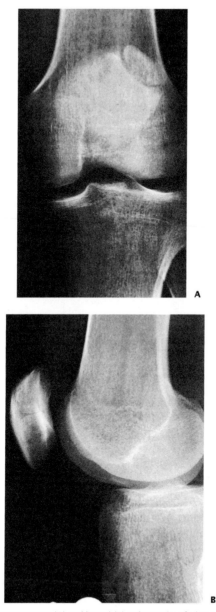

Figure 2   Anteroposterior **(A)** and lateral **(B)** radiographs of a bipartite patella. Note the superolateral fragment with well-defined cortical margins.

WHEN TO REFER

Open or displaced fractures require surgery. Referral to an orthopedist is needed if the patient is not progressing well with rehabilitation or if the fracture displaces while being treated in the cast.

COMPLICATIONS

Patellar fractures usually heal uneventfully. Possible complications include decreased range of motion, stiffness, fracture malunion, nonunion, and post-traumatic arthritis.

Chapter 8

FIBULAR FRACTURES

Manish K. Gupta and Robert L. Kalb

The fibula contributes only 15% of weight bearing in the lower extremity. Fractures of the fibula are common, especially with ankle injuries (Fig. 1).

MECHANISM OF INJURY

Isolated fibula fractures occur in three locations: (a) proximal fibula fracture due to an avulsion injury of the fibular collateral ligament secondary to a twisting of the knee, (b) distal fracture associated with an ankle syndesmotic injury due to twisting of the ankle, and (c) fracture of the fibula shaft due to a direct blow, such as a football helmet striking the lateral side of the leg.

DIAGNOSIS

The history of injury directs the physical examination, which shows point tenderness along the shaft of the fibula if fractured. If a proximal fibula fracture is present, examine the function of the peroneal nerve, which wraps around the fibular neck. In twisting injury of the ankle, examine the medial and lateral ankle for point tenderness. Plain radiographs include anteroposterior/lateral/mortise views of the ankle. If there is tenderness of the fibula proximally, then full-length anteroposterior/lateral tibia views are warranted.

INITIAL TREATMENT

If a fracture dislocation has occurred at the ankle, reduction with sedation is necessary followed by a posterior long-leg splint. If the fracture is localized to the proximal fibula, then ice, elevation, and a knee immobilizer are sufficient. Do not use an Ace wrap compression dressing on the leg. It can cause blood clots and edema. For a nondisplaced distal fibula fracture that does not disrupt the mortise (no widening of medial clear space due to lateral displacement of the talus), a short-leg splint, ice, and elevation, without weight bearing, are best.

DEFINITIVE TREATMENT

Treat a fibular fracture with a short-leg cast for 6 weeks. Follow-up for all patients should be every 2 weeks with x-rays until the fracture heals at 6 weeks. Full weight bearing begins in the walking cast at 3 weeks. Rehabilitation includes therapy to strengthen and to recover flexibility and proprioception.

WHEN TO REFER

With all fracture dislocations, surgery is necessary. Fractures with any medial space (mortise) widening of 2 mm or more require surgery (Fig. 2).

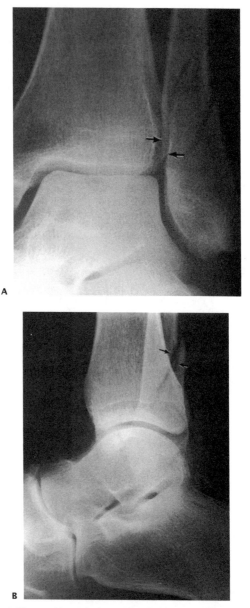

A

B

Figure 1 A 49-year-old prosthetist sustained a twisting injury to his ankle. Physical examination showed no medial swelling or tenderness. Mortise **(A)** and lateral **(B)** radiographs show fracture of the distal fibula with 2 mm lateral and posterior displacement (*arrows*). (*continues*)

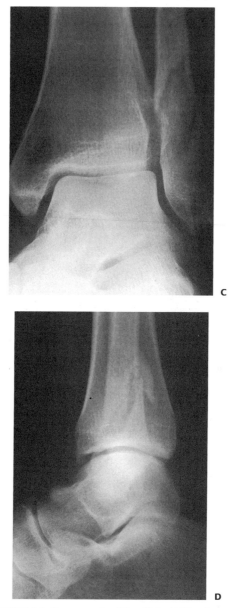

Figure 1 *Continued.* Follow-up mortise **(C)** and lateral **(D)** radiographs taken at 4 months after the injury demonstrate a stable mortise.

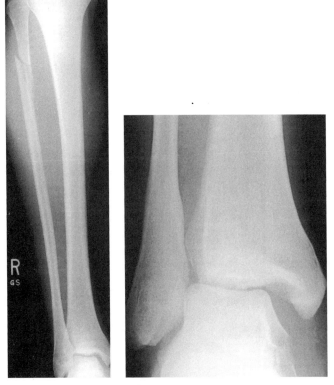

Figure 2   An anteroposterior radiograph of the tibia and fibula **(A)** shows a proximal fibula fracture without obvious shift of the talus. An external rotation stress view **(B)** shows significant widening of the medial clear space, lateral shift of the talus, and distal tibiofibular diastasis indicating an unstable injury.

COMPLICATIONS

Complications include nonunion, malunion, instability, stiffness, and complex regional pain syndrome. These complications are always more common in smokers.

Chapter 9

TIBIAL FRACTURES

Manish K. Gupta and Robert L. Kalb

TIBIAL PLATEAU FRACTURE

Fractures of the tibial plateau involve the articular surfaces of the proximal tibia that support the weight of the femoral condyles. These are serious injuries that can lead to functional impairment if not treated properly. Fractures can involve the medial or lateral plateau, or both. The goal is to maintain articular congruity, joint stability, and normal mechanical axis. This fracture is common in younger males due to high-energy trauma and in older osteoporotic females due to low-energy trauma.

Mechanism of Injury

Fracture of the tibial plateau occurs as a result of strong valgus or varus forces combined with axial loading. These occur with falls, sports injuries, and motor vehicle accidents. The typical "bumper" fracture occurs when the bumper of a car hits the lateral side of the knee. A valgus load is applied to the knee, and the lateral femoral condyle loads the lateral plateau, creating a fracture.

Diagnosis

The patient presents with pain and swelling of the knee and is unable to bear weight on the affected extremity. On physical examination, the patient has limited range of motion. A complete neurovascular assessment is done by checking distal pedal pulses and the function of the peroneal and tibial nerves of the involved extremity. The compartments of the leg should also be examined to rule out compartment syndrome. This is done by checking the tension of the skin, eliciting pain with passive extension of the big toe, and noting decreased light touch sensation in the first web space. If compartment syndrome is suspected, an orthopedic consultation is mandatory.

Radiology

Anteroposterior (AP)/lateral and a 20-degree caudal tilt AP x-ray are helpful. Fractures are classified according to where the fracture line extends (Fig. 1). In the past, treatment guidelines were based solely on x-ray; now, computed tomography scans are also used to assess articular depression and comminution.

Initial Treatment

The involved extremity is immobilized in a long posterior splint or immobilizer. All lacerations are cleaned and dressed. The extremity is elevated and iced. All displaced fractures of the tibial plateau require an orthopedic consultation for definitive care.

Definitive Treatment

If the fracture is nondisplaced and there is no concern of compartment syndrome, then the fracture can be treated in cast or knee immobilizer with non–weight bearing for 2 months. Rehabilitation goals are to recover strength and gain full range of motion. The patient should remove the brace daily for knee motion.

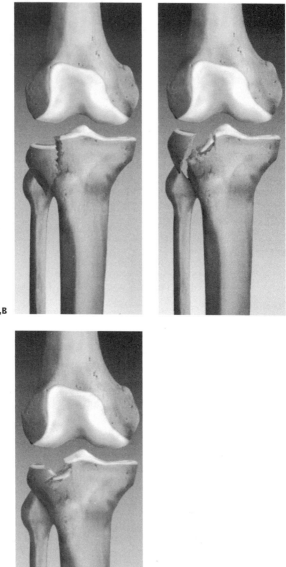

A,B

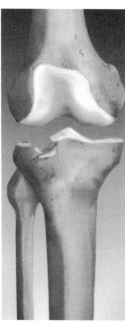

C

Figure 1 The Schatzker classification of tibial plateau fractures: type I **(A)**, type II **(B)**, and type III **(C)**.

When to Refer

If x-ray or computed tomography scans show greater than 3 mm of articular incongruity, surgery is recommended.

Complications

If these fractures are not treated properly, malalignment, early arthritis, and decreased function of the leg could occur.

TIBIAL SHAFT FRACTURES

Fractures of the tibial shaft are the most common long-bone fractures. Tibia fractures can be in the proximal, middle, and distal shafts of the tibia. These fractures constitute a spectrum of injuries that result in a loss of unrestricted load bearing of the extremity. This includes stress fractures, stable nondisplaced fractures from low-energy trauma, and extreme energy-absorbing injures that result in the loss of soft tissue, neurologic dysfunction, vascular insufficiency, and loss of bone. These could result in amputation.

Mechanism of Injury

Tibial shaft fractures result from three mechanisms: (a) torsional force injuries, in which the foot becomes fixed and the body rotates about the fixed point, as in a skiing injury; (b) three-point bending force injuries, which create short oblique or transverse fractures; and (c) direct blow injuries, which cause severe damage to the bone and soft tissues.

Diagnosis

The patient presents with pain, swelling, and inability to move the affected extremity. Because the tibia is subcutaneous, inspection of the overlying soft tissue is important to determine if the fracture is open or not. It is important to evaluate the pulses of the extremity and also to document the status of the peroneal nerve. Signs and symptoms of compartment syndrome should also be assessed.

Radiology

Standard AP/lateral full-length films of the tibia are all that is needed to evaluate. Bone scan or magnetic resonance imaging can be used to diagnose stress fractures of the tibia. Findings on x-ray can classify the fracture as a mild, moderate, or severe fracture with respect to soft tissue injury (Fig. 2).

Initial Treatment

The fracture is managed in a long-leg posterior splint, with ice and elevation. If there is gross deformity, the fracture should be reduced with traction under sedation and placed in a long posterior splint. An orthopedic evaluation is needed if the fracture is open and also if the fracture has more than 5 degrees of varus/valgus angulation on the AP view, or more than 10 degrees of angulation in a lateral view, more than 1 cm of shortening, or more than 50% displacement.

Definitive Treatment

If the fracture is nondisplaced or within the acceptable parameters of angulation and shortening, it can be treated closed in a long-leg cast. Follow-up is at 1 week initially, and then every 2 weeks until fracture union occurs in 3 months. The patient should be non–weight bearing. For stress fractures, the treatment is non–weight bearing. If the pain persists, the patient is placed in a cast. Rehabilitation goals are to gain full strength and function of the fractured extremity.

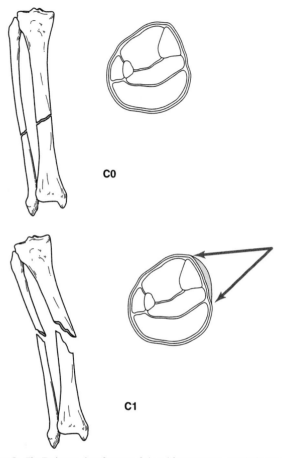

Figure 2 The Tscherne classification of closed fractures: C0, simple fracture configuration with little or no soft tissue injury. C1, superficial abrasion, mild to moderately severe fracture configuration. (*continues*).

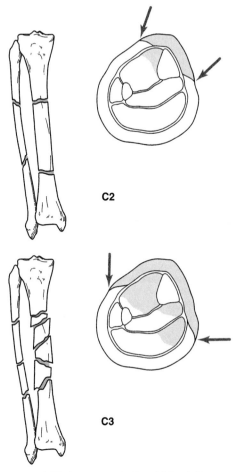

Figure 2 *Continued.* C2, deep contamination with local skin or muscle contusion, moderately severe fracture configuration. C3, extensive contusion or crushing of skin or destruction of muscle, severe fracture.

When to Refer

Fractures that are open, unstable, angulated, or shortened beyond acceptable standards need surgery.

Complications

The most common complications seen are nonunion, malunion, compartment syndrome, and leg length discrepancy.

Chapter 10

ANKLE FRACTURES

Arthur W. Pallotta and Robert L. Kalb

The incidence of ankle fractures has dramatically increased since the 1950s and approaches 150 per 100,000 persons. The incidence increases with age, particularly in women. Additional risk factors include obesity and history of smoking. The most common ankle fractures are isolated malleolar fractures, accounting for two-thirds of fractures, with bimalleolar fractures occurring in 25% and trimalleolar fractures in the remaining 7%. Open fractures are relatively rare, accounting for approximately 2% of all ankle fractures.

MECHANISM OF INJURY

History of a foot inversion with flexion (most common mechanism) involves the lateral ankle (distal fibular avulsion fracture). Eversion forces with dorsiflexion avulse the medial malleolus.

DIAGNOSIS

Ankle fractures are associated with pain, swelling, tenderness, and ecchymosis in association with point tenderness over the medial or lateral malleolus. Ankle fractures can be differentiated from sprains by the physical finding of point tenderness over the lateral malleolus (distal fibula) or medial malleolus. If there is no point tenderness over the malleoli, an x-ray is not necessary. Point tenderness over the lateral ligaments (anterior talofibular and calcaneal fibular ligament) is indicative of an ankle sprain. A first-degree ankle sprain has tenderness only over the anterior talofibular ligament, whereas a second- or third-degree ankle sprain has tenderness over the anterior talofibular ligament and the calcaneal fibular ligament, which lies more posterior.

RADIOLOGY

Three views are required: anteroposterior, lateral, and mortise. The mortise is an oblique view with the foot in approximately 15 degrees of internal rotation. There are three main types of distal fibular fractures: Weber types A, B, and C. The *Weber type A fracture* occurs below the level of the ankle mortise. (The ankle mortise is the joint space on the mortise view x-ray between the top of the talus and bottom of the tibia.) The *Weber type B fibular fracture* occurs at the level of the ankle mortise. The *Weber type C distal fibular fracture* occurs above the ankle mortise. Increased distance between the talus and the medial malleolus is sometimes seen (Fig. 1).

INITIAL TREATMENT

Reduce any associated dislocation immediately. Then elevate, ice, and splint, followed by non–weight bearing.

Medial Malleolar Fractures

If the fracture is nondisplaced, apply a short-leg cast. The ankle must be monitored closely for maintenance of reduction. Maintain non–weight bearing until there is radiographic evidence of healing at 3 weeks.

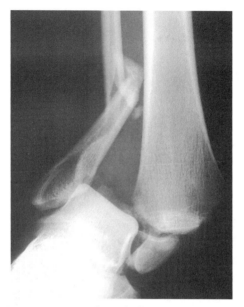

Figure 1 An anteroposterior radiograph of a typical pronation-abduction ankle fracture. The fibula is laterally comminuted.

Lateral Malleolar Fractures

Weber type A fractures can be treated immediately with a weight-bearing short-leg cast for 6 weeks. Nondisplaced Weber type B fractures can be treated with a short-leg walking cast for 6 weeks. The first 2 weeks must be non–weight bearing.

The Weber type C fracture (Fig. 2) has a greater potential for displacement and includes a portion of the syndesmotic ligament between the tibia and fibula just above the ankle mortise. Surgery is needed if any mortise widening occurs. If the syndesmosis is intact, this fracture can be treated with a walking cast for 6 weeks, but the first 3 weeks should be non–weight bearing. A cast boot prevents many of the complications of casts, such as toe injuries and skin breakdown from foreign bodies introduced under the cast (Fig. 2).

With all lateral malleolar fractures, it is important to rule out medial injury. Although the x-ray may be negative for a medial fracture, tenderness medially with a lateral fracture indicates an unstable ankle (termed *bimalleolar equivalent*). This changes the patient's weight-bearing status to non–weight bearing and requires surgery if the mortise is widened on the mortise view.

DEFINITIVE TREATMENT

Medial and lateral malleolar fractures require a minimum of 6 weeks for healing. If the patient smokes, or has a history of poorly controlled diabetes, the fracture healing time can double. Restore anatomic alignment at the ankle to

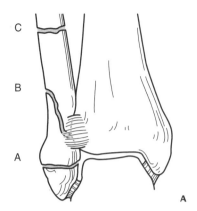

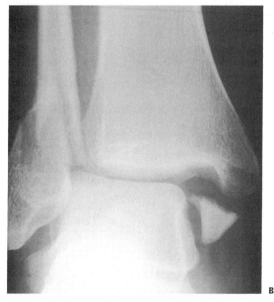

Figure 2 Schematic diagram and case examples of the classification of ankle fractures. **A:** There are three types: type A, type B, and type C. **B:** An anteroposterior radiograph of a type A distal fibula fracture in which the fracture line is completely below the level of the syndesmosis. (*continues*)

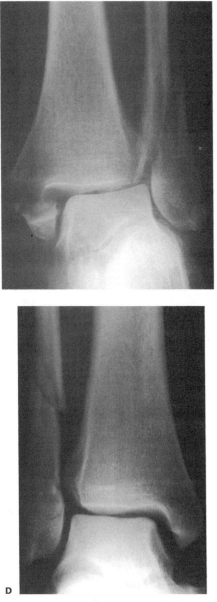

Figure 2 *Continued.* **C:** A radiograph of a type B ankle fracture in which the fibula fracture begins anteriorly at the distal tibiofibular level of the fibula fracture, which is completely above the distal syndesmotic ligament complex. **D:** There is a medial deltoid ligament injury. Note the widened medial joint space as the talus shifted laterally.

minimize osteoarthritis, maximize future stability, and give the best chance at returning to the preinjury lifestyle. Goals include restoring range of motion, recovering proprioception, and achieving ankle control by strengthening.

WHEN TO REFER

Any displaced intraarticular fracture, displaced bimalleolar fracture (unstable), or open fracture and any fracture in which the mortise is widened should be referred.

COMPLICATIONS

Fracture union is delayed for people who smoke or use ibuprofen. The incidence of reflex sympathetic dystrophy is much greater in smokers. Stiffness in a joint is increased in diabetics or smokers. Patients can better appreciate this when they understand that diabetes and smoking both decrease capillary blood flow.

Chapter 11

FOOT FRACTURES

Arthur W. Pallotta and Robert L. Kalb

TALUS FRACTURES

During the Second World War, the foot controls of airplane landing gear were mechanical. Sometimes, these controls would snap back suddenly into the sole of the foot of the pilot, resulting in axial loading of the talus and a fracture. During that time, the talus fracture became known as *aviator's astragalus* (Fig. 1).

Mechanism of Injury

The talus can fracture with a sudden axial loading on the foot, most commonly with dorsiflexion (Fig. 2).

Diagnosis

The symptoms of talus fracture are similar to those of an ankle fracture.

Radiology

Anteroposterior (AP), lateral, and oblique views of the foot should be obtained along with AP, lateral, and mortise (discussed in Chapter 10) views of the ankle.

Initial Treatment

Emergent treatment is instrumental in preserving neurologic and vascular function. If dislocation is present, an immediate reduction is indicated. If the dislocation cannot be reduced, emergent open reduction is indicated to decrease the chance of avascular necrosis.

Definitive Treatment

The definitive goal is to obtain the best possible reduction and to protect the reduction. This gives the best chance at union and reduces the incidence of posttraumatic arthritis. The risk of avascular necrosis is proportional to the original amount of displacement. If the fracture is nondisplaced, use a short-leg cast for 6 weeks, non–weight bearing, followed by an additional 6 weeks of weight bearing in the cast.

When to Refer

Any talus fracture that is displaced should be seen by an orthopedist that day.

Complications

Patients should be informed that there is a high incidence of osteoarthritis, as well as avascular necrosis. Talus fracture complications are as common as those in the scaphoid.

CALCANEUS FRACTURES

The most common mechanism for calcaneus fracture (axial loading) often produces concomitant thoracic and lumbar compression fractures.

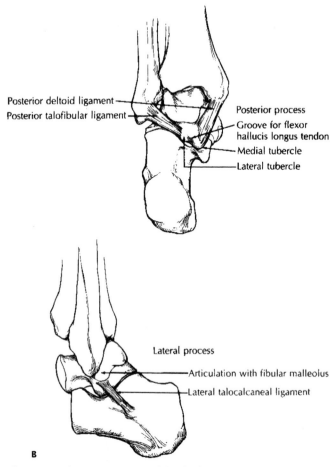

Posterior deltoid ligament
Posterior talofibular ligament

Posterior process
Groove for flexor hallucis longus tendon
Medial tubercle
Lateral tubercle

A

Lateral process
Articulation with fibular malleolus
Lateral talocalcaneal ligament

B

Figure 1   A: The posterior process of the talus has two tubercles, which are separated by the groove for the flexor hallucis longus tendon. The posterior fibers of the deltoid ligament insert into the medial tubercle, and the posterior talofibular ligament inserts into the lateral tubercle. **B:** The lateral process of the talus.

Mechanism of Injury

The calcaneus can be fractured as a result of a fall from a height, jumpers' injuries, or a direct blow striking the posterior calcaneus.

Diagnosis

History of fall from a height with pain in the heel or tenderness over the medial, lateral, or plantar surface of the calcaneus should raise suspicion. It is usually accompanied by ecchymosis, swelling, and pain with weight bearing. Palpate thoracic and lumbar spinous processes for associated injuries.

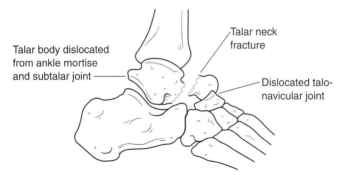

Figure 2   Talar neck fracture. Note that, in addition to the displacement of the talar body with subluxation of the subtalar joint, the talonavicular joint is also dislocated.

Radiology

AP, lateral, and oblique views of the foot should be obtained, as well as an axial view of the calcaneus (Fig. 3). Computed tomography is often necessary to evaluate the articular surfaces. Thoracic and lumbar spine films to aid in ruling out associated compression fractures should be done if tenderness is noted.

Initial Treatment

Initial treatment consists of ice and elevation, with the hip and knee flexed at 90 degrees each to keep the heel at least 2 feet higher than the heart at all times, for 2 weeks. Avoid splint or cast.

Definitive Treatment

As with talus fractures, the definitive goal is to obtain the best possible reduction, protect the reduction, and correct any intraarticular displacement of the fracture. Whether surgery is performed or not, these fractures require 3 months of non–weight bearing.

When to Refer

Patients with any displaced fracture in the calcaneus should be referred. A computed tomography scan should be done immediately to determine the extent of intraarticular displacement, so that surgical treatment options can be considered. Always check for thoracic and lumbar spine fracture, which can often accompany fracture of the calcaneus because of the same axial-loading mechanism of injury for both. If there is any doubt about displacement, you should consult a radiologist or an orthopedist. Maximal elevation is critical to minimize swelling and pain. Elevation with the patient lying down and the hip and knee flexed to 90 degrees with couch cushions under the calf is best at all times for the first week. Flexing both the hip and the knee decreases the stretch on the sciatic nerve; this decreases the incidence of sciatica.

Complications

The most common complication is posttraumatic subtalar arthritis, which results in decreased range of subtalar eversion and inversion.

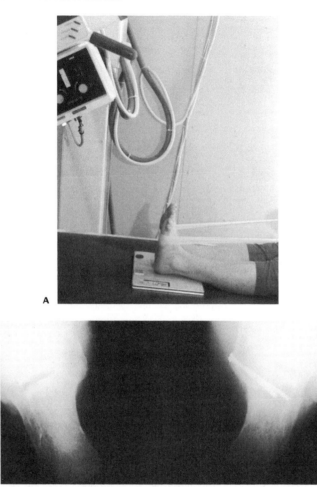

Figure 3 **A:** Photograph of the radiographic technique for obtaining the Harris or calcaneal radiographic view. Maximum dorsiflexion of the ankle was attempted to obtain an optimal view. **B:** Calcaneal views of bilateral calcanei. Normal is on the left; intraarticular fixation of sustentaculum fracture is on the right.

MIDFOOT TARSAL FRACTURES

The midfoot tarsal bones include the cuneiforms, cuboid, and navicular.

Mechanism of Injury

Tarsal fractures can occur as a result of indirect trauma (torsion) or direct trauma.

Diagnosis

Pain and swelling with tenderness in the midfoot should raise suspicion.

Radiology

AP, lateral, and oblique views of the foot should be obtained. Computed tomography can further evaluate any fracture that cannot be fully characterized by plain films.

Initial Treatment

As in other fractures, ice and elevation are important acutely.

Definitive Treatment

Nondisplaced fractures are treated appropriately in a short-leg cast, non–weight bearing for 6 weeks.

When to Refer

If the fracture is displaced, refer to an orthopedist. For fractures extending into the tarsometatarsal joint, look for a tarsometatarsal dislocation. This joint is also referred to as the *Lisfranc joint*. All three x-ray views of the foot are important in evaluation of this rare but serious injury. If you have any questions about fracture in the midfoot, have an orthopedic surgeon or radiologist review the films with you.

Complications

For fractures at this level, the most common complications are osteoarthritis and osteonecrosis.

METATARSAL FRACTURES

Metatarsal fractures are very common in the foot; be suspicious with direct-blow or twisting injuries.

Mechanism of Injury

Metatarsals can be fractured as a result of various mechanisms. Axial-loading, crushing force, and twisting injuries are all common. Motor vehicle accidents with a sudden deceleration are a common mechanism. Stress fractures in runners are also common.

Diagnosis

Swelling and tenderness in the foot along with a history of trauma should raise suspicion for these fractures. Open fractures, skin tenting, and blanching secondary to pressure from displaced fractures are dangerous signs.

Radiology

AP, lateral, and oblique radiographs of the foot should be obtained.

Initial Treatment

Compartment syndrome can occur in the foot. It occurs most often with multiple metatarsal fractures, although it is much less common than in the forearm or the calf. Elevation, ice, and splint immobilization improve comfort. Initially, a posterior splint and non–weight bearing are appropriate treatment.

Definitive Treatment

In cases with severe swelling, the splint should be changed to a short-leg walking cast once the swelling has subsided.

Non- or minimally (<2 mm) displaced fractures of the metatarsals at the shaft level may be treated in a short-leg walking cast. The patient should be weight bearing as tolerated in a short-leg cast for 5 weeks.

When to Refer

Displaced fractures of the metatarsals should be referred, as well as fractures of multiple metatarsals. Any indication of compartment syndrome or any displacement at the tarsometatarsal joint on the AP, lateral, or oblique views of the foot is a reason to obtain an orthopedic consult urgently. A greater-than-5-mm displaced avulsion fracture of the base of the fifth metatarsal should be referred (Fig. 4A).

Fracture of the proximal one-third of the shaft of the fifth metatarsal, associated with displacement, requires special attention. It is important to differentiate an avulsion of the base of the fifth metatarsal from a true Jones fracture (Fig. 4B), which is much less common but is treated differently. The true Jones fracture extends across the entire proximal shaft. If the fracture is displaced, the patient should be referred to an orthopedist. If it is nondis-

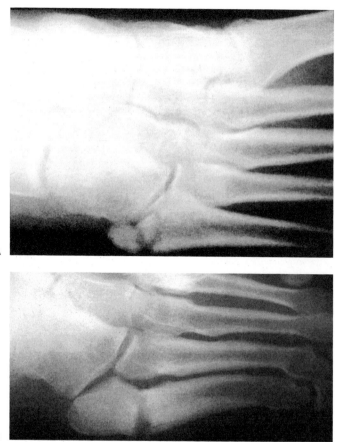

A

B

Figure 4   A: Fracture of the fifth metatarsal base. **B:** True Jones fracture.

placed, the patient should wear a short-leg cast, non–weight bearing, for 6 weeks. Then a walking cast is used for 6 weeks. This fracture is notorious for delayed union, especially in patients who smoke or take antiinflammatory medication. Ibuprofen delays fracture union. In displaced fractures, the non-union rate is high. Patients should not participate in sports for at least 3 months.

Complications

With multiple fractures of three or more metatarsals from a crushing-type injury, extreme swelling can occur. This may require decompression for compartment syndrome. It is rare but can occur. Multiple metatarsal fractures must be treated similarly to calcaneal fractures: 90-degree hip and knee flexion position and elevation with four couch cushions under the calf at all times for 1 week. Malunion may result in metatarsal overload syndrome due to unequal load sharing of the metatarsal heads.

TOE FRACTURES

Toe fractures are underdiagnosed, and great-toe fractures require special consideration.

Mechanism of Injury

Toe fractures are most commonly due to direct axial load due to stubbing the toe or crush injury.

Diagnosis

Toe fractures cause pain, swelling, and point tenderness. Also, nail-plate injury, ecchymosis, or deformity suggests fracture.

Radiology

AP, lateral, and oblique views of the involved toe should be obtained.

Initial Treatment

Ice and elevation can help reduce swelling. Any malrotation deformity should be corrected. Displaced fractures can be managed well by reduction aided by a digital block and traction, pulling the toe into a corrected position, followed by buddy taping for 3 weeks or using a wooden-sole shoe, or both. Buddy taping stabilizes the toe and makes the patient more comfortable. When taping digits together, place dry cotton between the digits to prevent skin maceration from moisture. Patients can change their dressing after a shower. Three to four weeks is the recommended duration of treatment.

Definitive Treatment

Whether in the operating room or in the office, the goal is to achieve union with an acceptable reduction.

When to Refer

Any intraarticular displaced or open fracture of the great toe should be referred to an orthopedist.

Fractures in the fingers or toes sometimes involve injury to the nail bed caused by the bone pushing up. Treatment should include using a digital block anesthetic and removal of the nail to thoroughly irrigate the nail bed at the site of the open fracture. The nail bed can be repaired with 5-0 Vicryl suture. Repair helps to prevent nail deformity. Nail-bed repair is more appropriate for fingers than for toes. Most people do not mind some deformity of the toe nail plate but have more cosmetic concern when it occurs in the finger.

Complications

Nonunion and posttraumatic arthritis are the most frequent complications. Posttraumatic arthritis can be disabling if it involves the great toe.

Chapter 12

CLAVICULAR FRACTURES

David V. Lopez and Robert L. Kalb

The clavicle is one of the most frequently injured bones. Fractures are classified according to their location in the middle, lateral, or medial third.

MECHANISM OF INJURY

By a direct blow, the clavicle can be fractured in contact sport, by motor vehicle accident, or by newborn birth trauma from shoulder dystocia.

DIAGNOSIS

Common findings include swelling, deformity, and point tenderness over the clavicle, which is subcutaneous and easily palpable.

Always listen to the chest to make sure there is no pneumothorax related to the clavicle fracture, especially for those fractures caused by motor vehicle accidents. Instruct the patient to let you know immediately if he or she has any shortness of breath.

RADIOLOGY

Radiographic imaging includes anteroposterior as well as cephalic and caudal tilt views to assess displacement.

INITIAL TREATMENT

Treatment is symptomatic and includes a figure-of-eight brace or sling, both, or neither, depending on the patient's comfort level. If the patient is comfortable in the sling, then a figure-of-eight brace is not needed if the clavicle fracture is nondisplaced. The goal is to restore anatomic alignment and length of the clavicle. If the clavicle fracture is overriding (bayonet position), reduction is necessary with a figure-of-eight splint. If this is not done, the fracture will heal with a shortening. This results in foreshortening of the shoulder and poor cosmesis.

DEFINITIVE TREATMENT

Almost all clavicle fractures are treated closed, and only on rare occasions is operative intervention required. Most often, a sling is satisfactory. A figure-of-eight splint is indicated in cases of bayonet apposition. With the patient seated, adjust the figure-of-eight splint so that it is tight enough to be supportive but yet not so tight that it causes tingling and numbness from pressure on the brachial plexus as the splint wraps around the armpit. The patient can tighten the brace daily to maintain support. The brace or sling is worn for 6 weeks. Clavicle fractures require a minimum of 2 months for solid union (Fig. 1), and contact sports should be avoided for 3 months after the fracture. Inform patients that as healing progresses, there may be a prominent callus; this usually resorbs with time. Rehabilitation goals include recovering range of motion and strength in the shoulder by means of physical therapy in adults if function is not normal with activities of daily living.

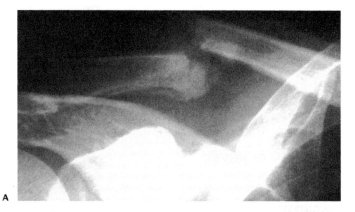

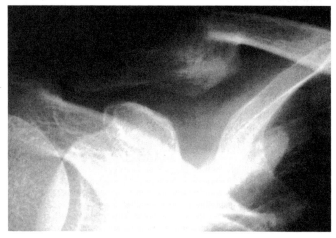

Figure 1 Typical midclavicle fracture **(A)**, which went on to uneventful healing with closed treatment **(B)**.

WHEN TO REFER

Severe overriding bayonet apposition that cannot be reduced by application of a figure-of-eight clavicle strap and tenting of the skin by the sharp clavicle fracture fragment to the point that the skin is void of circulation and therefore at risk for necrosis reduction should be referred.

COMPLICATIONS

The clavicle is the only bony connection of the entire shoulder girdle to the skeleton. If the clavicle heals in a bayonet position, the shoulder will be close to the midline. This may be cosmetically significant. Fractures involving the lateral third of the clavicle may develop a nonunion or symptomatic acromioclavicular joint arthritis. A painful nonunion (no radiographic healing after 4 to 6 months) may need operative management. This is rare; most nonunions are not painful.

Chapter 13

SCAPULAR FRACTURES

David V. Lopez and Robert L. Kalb

Fractures of the scapula represent an uncommon injury. The rib cage, thick soft tissue covering, and its mobility help to explain this. The anatomic regions that may be injured include the scapula body and spine, glenoid neck, glenoid cavity (Fig. 1), and the acromial and coracoid processes.

MECHANISM OF INJURY

Scapula fractures are usually caused by high-energy trauma. Direct forces are most often the cause, although indirect mechanisms, such as a fall on the arm, may produce a fracture. There is a high incidence of associated injuries.

DIAGNOSIS

Pain, tenderness, swelling, and ecchymosis are the first clues.

RADIOLOGY

Radiographic evaluations should include scapular true anteroposterior and true lateral views.

INITIAL TREATMENT

The scapula fracture is immobilized in a sling and swathe.

DEFINITIVE TREATMENT

Once other injuries have been excluded or managed, attention may be directed to the scapula fracture. Sling and swathe immobilization is satisfactory. Once pain subsides, pendulum exercises, along with elbow and hand range of motion, are initiated. Radiographs are taken to ensure that unacceptable displacement does not occur. By 6 weeks, most fractures have healed, and external immobilization is discontinued. Progressive range of motion and strengthening are undertaken.

WHEN TO REFER

In the event of a rare open or displaced intraarticular fracture, refer. Nondisplaced intraarticular glenoid and glenoid neck fractures do not need to be referred.

COMPLICATIONS

The early complications may include neurovascular injuries. Later issues may include restricted shoulder motion after the injury.

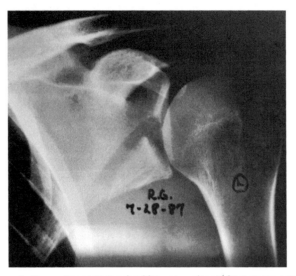

Figure 1 True anteroposterior shoulder x-ray—glenoid fracture requiring fixation.

Chapter 14

HUMERAL FRACTURES

David V. Lopez and Robert L. Kalb

Shoulder (glenohumeral) dislocations and fractures account for the majority of injuries about the shoulder girdle. The proximal humerus parts are the articular surface, anatomic neck, greater and lesser tuberosities, surgical neck, and the proximal portion of the diaphysis. The humeral diaphysis begins from the proximal border of the insertion of the pectoralis major and ends distally at the supracondylar ridge.

GLENOHUMERAL DISLOCATIONS

Mechanism of Injury

Glenohumeral dislocations may be either anterior or posterior. Anterior dislocations (90%) result from a direct posterior blow or abduction and external rotation of the shoulder. Posterior dislocations (10%) result from seizures, direct anterior force, or adduction and axial loading of the arm.

Diagnosis

A concavity at the glenoid fossa is noted. The patient is unable to elevate the arm to the head area. A neurovascular examination is done to determine any deficits. Shoulder dislocation may affect the brachial plexus or axillary nerve. Anterior dislocation patients hold the arm in external rotation. With posterior dislocations, the arm is held in internal rotation and adduction.

Radiology

A true anteroposterior (AP) view and scapula views should be taken. The true AP view should display overlap of the anterior and posterior articular surface of the glenoid. The view should show the humerus head centered on the glenoid.

Initial Treatment

Conscious sedation is often necessary to reduce a dislocated shoulder. The sooner the shoulder is reduced, the easier it is. Straight traction in line with the humerus with gentle internal and external rotation reduces the dislocation. This reduction method is safe even if a fracture is present. It is necessary to apply countertraction via a sheet wrapped around the chest wall. The shoulder is abducted 30 degrees for the reduction. After a neurovascular examination, immobilization is carried out in a shoulder immobilizer or sling and swathe.

It is standard care to reduce a shoulder dislocation as an emergency even if the patient has just eaten. The longer the shoulder is dislocated, the higher the incidence of avascular necrosis.

Definitive Treatment

Uncomplicated dislocations are immobilized for 3 weeks, beginning isometrics immediately. Patients younger than 18 years of age should be referred to an orthopedist on the first dislocation. This is due to potential growth plate injury and high rate of recurrence.

When to Refer

A vascular compromise is an emergency and should be surgically addressed immediately. Dislocations associated with fractures of the head or diaphysis, or both, should be seen by an orthopedist. Also, dislocations more than a day or two old or a recurrent dislocation should be managed by an orthopedist.

Complications

Complications may include stiffness and rotator cuff tears, which may be surgically treated. The axillary nerve may be injured. Signs include loss of light touch over the lateral shoulder, where the skin in a silver dollar–sized area is supplied by sensory branches only from the axillary nerve. Another sign of axillary neuropraxia is inferior subluxation of the shoulder on the AP x-ray after reduction. This is due to the deltoid upward pull on the humerus being absent until the nerve recovers. It almost always recovers.

FRACTURES OF THE PROXIMAL HUMERUS

Mechanism of Injury

Fractures of the proximal humerus often result from an impact to the shoulder from a low-energy fall in the elderly or from high-energy trauma in the young. A dislocation may occur concurrently.

Diagnosis

On visual inspection, there is swelling and possibly ecchymosis. Most often, the fracture involves some combination of the anatomic neck, the surgical neck, the greater tuberosity, and the lesser tuberosity. The fracture may be categorized into one of three groups: two-part, three-part, and four-part fractures.

Radiology

True AP and true lateral (scapula Y) radiographs of the shoulder should be obtained.

Initial Treatment

All injuries may be initially placed in a sling and swathe with ice. Fractures of the greater tuberosity with displacement of less than 1.0 cm and angulation of less than 45 degrees (Fig. 1) are treated in a shoulder immobilizer (Table 1).

Definitive Treatment

Pendulum exercise is begun at 3 weeks, and more aggressive strengthening is begun at 6 weeks and continued for 6 months. Two-part surgical neck fractures may be reduced under conscious sedation. Traction is applied to the arm with flexion and adduction while attempting to correct the angulation. Once reduced, the elbow is pushed upward, like jamming a mushroom stem up into the cap, and the arm is placed in a sling and swathe. Immobilization should take place for 3 weeks before beginning pendulum exercises. At 6 weeks, gentle active resistive exercises are initiated.

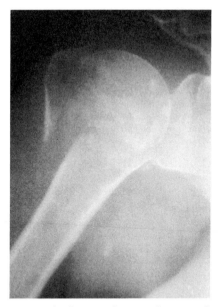

Figure 1 Despite several millimeters of greater tuberosity and surgical neck displacement, the patient gained full painless motion after nonoperative treatment.

When to Refer

Unstable reductions, any vascular (emergent) or neurologic compromise, and irreducible fractures should be seen by an orthopedist.

Complications

Complications include adhesive capsulitis (frozen shoulder). This even applies to patients with minimal displacement.

TABLE 1	Indications for Nonoperative Treatment
Nondisplaced fractures	<5 mm of superior or 10 mm of posterior greater tuberosity displacement in active people. <10 mm of superior displacement in nondominant arm of sedentary patients.
Surgical neck fractures	Any bone contact in elderly patients. In young, active patients, <50% shaft diameter displacement and <45-degree angulation in dominant arm.
Reduced demands	Patient willing to accept stiff shoulder.
Poor health	Patient unable to tolerate surgery and anesthesia.
Poor rehabilitation candidate	Patient too feeble to pursue rehabilitation or unable to understand or remember postoperative restrictions.

HUMERAL SHAFT FRACTURES

Mechanism of Injury

Humeral shaft fractures result from direct trauma or a torsional force, as in arm wrestling.

Diagnosis

Pain, swelling, and deformity often characterize the injury. As usual, a careful neurovascular examination is performed. Radial nerve injuries occur in up to 20% of humeral fractures. The physical findings include loss of dorsal thumb sensation and inability to extend the wrist or metacarpophalangeal joints.

Radiology

The radiographic examination includes AP and lateral radiographs. The fracture patterns include transverse, oblique, segmental, and comminuted.

Initial Treatment

Early stabilization includes aligning or reducing the fracture under sedation and placing a coaptation splint. The fracture is reduced with gravity and traction downward. Then the splint starts from over the contralateral shoulder, across the back of the neck, over the shoulder, down the arm, and across the elbow in 90 degrees flexion, and to the mid-palm. A shoulder immobilizer then goes over it.

Definitive Treatment

Fractures that may need surgical management include open fractures; multiple trauma; injury of the brachial artery; segmental fractures; ipsilateral fractures and dislocations of the elbow, shoulder, and forearm; bilateral humeral shaft fractures; pathologic fractures; and failed closed reduction. Obese or uncooperative patients may also require surgical management. Limits of acceptable alignment are 20 degrees of AP angulation, 30 degrees of varus or valgus, and 3 cm of shortening. The coaptation splint can be maintained until union. Elbow motion begins at 3 weeks. At 6 weeks, a functional brace may be exchanged for the coaptation splint, with therapy starting at 6 weeks and advancing as tolerated. At the time of union, usually 12 weeks, the brace is discontinued (Fig. 2).

When to Refer

One should refer to an orthopedist if there is not union at 6 months postinjury. Other reasons to refer are for surgical management and unacceptable position.

Complications

Complications may include loss of reduction. If the radial nerve is working normally at presentation followed by wrist drop after splinting, remove the splint and refer. Surgery occurs emergently if wrist drop occurs after an attempted closed reduction. Surgery to explore the nerve is not indicated if wrist drop is present when the patient presents for treatment. Nonunion is another complication.

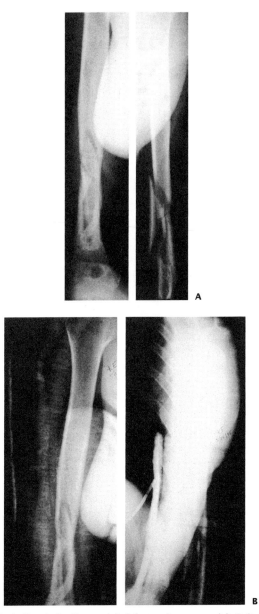

Figure 2   A: Closed, distal humeral shaft fracture in a young adult. **B:** Stabilized initially with a coaptation splint. Functional orthosis was placed 10 days after injury. (*continues*)

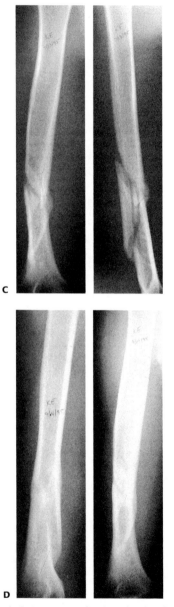

Figure 2 *Continued.* **C:** Appearance after 8 weeks when fracture was clinically united. **D:** Appearance 16 weeks after injury.

Chapter 15

ELBOW FRACTURES

David V. Lopez and Robert L. Kalb

The elbow consists of articulations of the distal humerus with the ulna and radius. The latter two articulate with each other to form the proximal radial ulnar joint. This chapter covers fractures of the distal humerus, the radial head, the olecranon, and the coronoid process and dislocations of the elbow.

FRACTURES OF THE DISTAL HUMERUS (SUPRACONDYLAR AND CONDYLAR FRACTURES)

Mechanism of Injury

A fall on an outstretched hand is common in the sporting and recreation settings, whereas a direct blow is more common in the occupational arena.

Diagnosis

There may be point tenderness pain, swelling, deformity, and instability of the elbow. As always, one should conduct a thorough neurovascular examination of the extremity.

Radiology

Anteroposterior, lateral, and oblique radiographs show the fracture. Computed tomography may be useful with condylar fractures. There is dissociation between the diaphysis and the humeral condyles with variable intercondylar extension (Fig. 1). Condylar fractures involve either the capitellum or the trochlea, or both.

Initial Treatment

The elbow should hang by the side and be immobilized with a posterior long-arm splint with the elbow flexed 90 degrees. A sling is used for support, and ice is used to decrease swelling.

Definitive Treatment

Fractures of the distal humerus require operative treatment if displaced. Refer displaced injuries for orthopedic evaluation.

When to Refer

Displaced fractures should be referred as well as any with neurovascular compromise.

Complications

Complications include stiffness, loss of motion, pain, malunion, and nonunion.

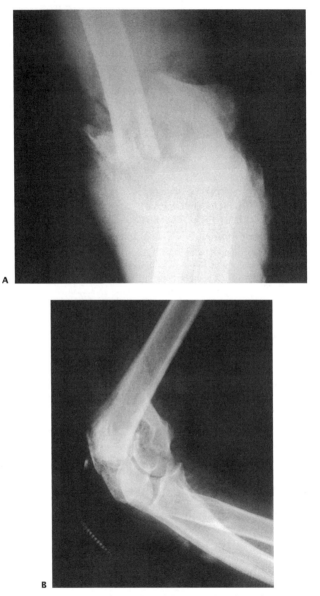

A

B

Figure 1   Anteroposterior **(A)** and lateral **(B)** x-rays that, due to bone overlap, poorly show the details of the fracture. (*continues*)

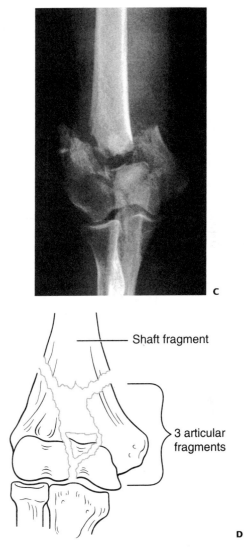

Shaft fragment

3 articular
fragments

C

D

Figure 1 *Continued.* A traction x-ray **(C)** nicely shows the important details of
the fracture and enables the surgeon to make a formal preoperative plan **(D)**.

FRACTURES OF THE RADIAL HEAD

Mechanism of Injury

Most commonly, fractures of the radial head result from a fall on an outstretched hand (Fig. 2).

Diagnosis

Tenderness localizes to the lateral side of the elbow.

Radiology

Radiographs should include anteroposterior, lateral, and oblique views. Forearm and wrist radiographs are done if tenderness is present. Fractures may be nondisplaced, displaced, comminuted (greater than two fragments), or associated with dislocation at the elbow or wrist.

Initial Treatment

Assess the elbow range of motion for a mechanical block in nondisplaced and partially displaced fractures. First, a hematoma can be aspirated from the radiocapitellar articulation. This is the center of a triangle formed from the bony landmarks of the lateral epicondyle, radial head, and olecranon. 10 ml of 1% lidocaine is infiltrated. Flexion/extension is normally 0 to 160 degrees with 90 degrees of pronation and 90 degrees of supination. Ligamentous testing with varus and valgus stress is done with the elbow flexed 15 degrees. Valgus instability indicates a torn medial collat-

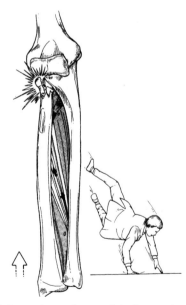

Figure 2 A fall that produces a fracture of the forearm also can strain or rupture the interosseous membrane.

eral ligament. Associated elbow dislocation should be reduced (see section Fracture Dislocations of the Elbow). Finally, the elbow is placed in a posterior splint at 120 degrees.

Definitive Treatment

Nondisplaced fractures are immobilized with a sling and long-arm splint only if they are too painful without. Displaced fractures without a mechanical block may be treated as nondisplaced fractures. The sooner motion is started, the less the chance of stiffness. Radial head fracture does not require a splint because the orbicular ligament holds it in place.

When to Refer

A block to motion may need operative treatment and should be referred. Comminuted fractures, wrist and forearm tenderness (possible Essex-Lopresti injury), and an unstable elbow should be splinted and referred.

Complications

Even with minimally displaced fractures, there may be a loss of several degrees of range of motion. This is not a problem because normal elbow function requires only a total of 100 degrees of range of motion.

FRACTURES OF THE OLECRANON

Mechanism of Injury

Fractures of the olecranon often result from a direct blow.

Diagnosis

Tenderness, swelling, and ecchymosis localize over the tip of the elbow. Anteroposterior and lateral radiographs of the elbow are sufficient (Fig. 3). To determine operative versus conservative treatment, one must assess the intraarticular displacement. Fractures may be treated conservatively when there is less than 2 mm of displacement and no increase in displacement with elbow flexion at 90 degrees.

Initial Treatment

The injured elbow is placed in a posterior splint at 20 degrees. Elevation and ice are encouraged to minimize swelling and discomfort.

Definitive Treatment

The nondisplaced, conservatively treated olecranon fracture may be placed in a posterior splint at 20 degrees for 4 weeks. Repeat x-rays are obtained at 7 to 10 days to ensure no displacement. A sling is used at 3 weeks, range of motion is begun, and the elbow is flexed to 90 degrees in a new splint. Maximal motion may not return for 6 to 12 months.

When to Refer

All displaced fractures should be referred to an orthopedic surgeon within a week.

Complications

Complications may include late displacement of a nondisplaced fracture, decreased flexion or extension, and articular damage from the impact at the time of injury.

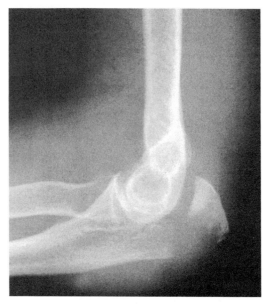

Figure 3 Fracture of the olecranon. Note the comminution and disruption of the articular surface; a true lateral view is necessary to visualize this adequately. The pull of the triceps tendon is the displacing force on the proximal fragment.

FRACTURE DISLOCATIONS OF THE ELBOW

Mechanism of Injury

Fracture dislocations of the elbow result from either a hyperextension injury or an axial load applied to a slightly flexed elbow.

Diagnosis

Pain and swelling are the predominant clinical findings. A careful neurovascular examination is important.

Radiology

Anteroposterior and lateral radiographs are essential, as associated fractures may exist or the injury may actually be a supracondylar fracture. The radius and ulna most often dislocate together posteriorly, medially, laterally, or anteriorly. Also, the coronoid may be fractured (Fig. 4).

Initial Treatment

Reduce the dislocation as soon as possible (Fig. 5). Conscious sedation is recommended to facilitate the maneuver. One applies traction to the forearm with simultaneous countertraction to the upper arm. The medial-lateral alignment is corrected before flexion of the elbow. The reduced elbow is brought through a full range of motion, and stability is tested with varus and valgus

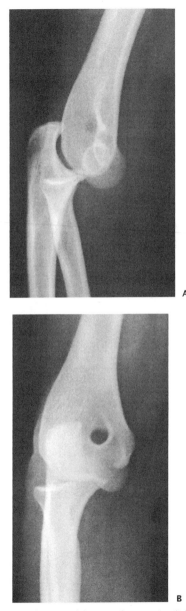

Figure 4 Lateral **(A)** and anterior **(B)** views of a posterior dislocation of the elbow, in which the coronoid is impaled into the trochlea. In this injury, the coronoid could fracture from the impact.

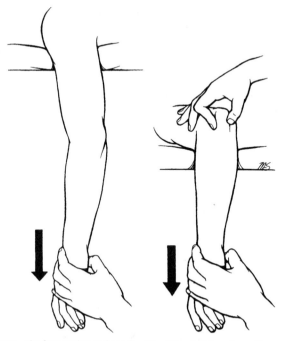

Figure 5   The forearm hangs from the side of the stretcher. As gentle downward traction is applied on the wrist, the physician guides reduction of the olecranon with the opposite hand. (Redrawn from Meyn MA, Quigley TB. Reduction of posterior dislocation of the elbow by traction on the dangling arm. *Clin Orthop* 1974;103:106–108.)

stress. The elbow is stabilized in a posterior splint at 120 degrees of flexion before postreduction radiographs are taken.

Definitive Treatment

Stable, reduced dislocations are immobilized for 3 weeks before initiating active range of motion in physical therapy. If the elbow is not kept in 120-degree flexion, the triceps tension to stabilize the elbow is less, and the elbow reduction may be lost.

When to Refer

Unstable dislocations with articular fractures, coronoid fractures involving more than its tip, irreducible dislocations, and suspected compartment syndromes (emergent) require care by an orthopedist.

Complications

Complications mostly consist of loss of motion. Heterotopic ossification (extraosseous bone formation) may be the cause. It is important to prevent passive-stretch elbow motion in adults or children because this may cause heterotopic ossification.

Chapter 16

FRACTURES OF THE FOREARM AND DISTAL RADIUS

David V. Lopez and Robert L. Kalb

The forearm consists of the radius and ulna shafts. Maintaining their anatomic relationship preserves pronation and supination. As a result, many fractures of the forearm require operative fixation. Also mentioned here are injuries to the distal radius.

FOREARM FRACTURES

Mechanism of Injury

A direct injury or a fall on an outstretched arm may precipitate an injury.

Diagnosis

Forearm fractures are associated with swelling, pain, and point tenderness. Neurovascular structures are intimately associated with the osseous structures in this area; a careful examination is important.

Radiology

Plain anteroposterior and lateral radiographs provide sufficient information for diagnosis and management (Fig. 1). There may be an isolated or both-bone fracture of the radius and ulna. The Monteggia fracture (Fig. 2) is a fracture of the proximal ulna with dislocation of the radial head. The Galeazzi fracture (Fig. 3) is a fracture of the distal third of the radius with dislocation or subluxation of the distal radioulnar joint.

Initial Treatment

With the exception of the isolated ulna fracture (nightstick fracture), all of these injuries are best immobilized using a long-arm posterior splint. Traction in fingertraps may be necessary to correct angulation. Isolated ulna shaft fractures with less than 50% displacement and 15 degrees of angulation may be managed nonoperatively. A long-arm posterior splint may be applied.

Definitive Treatment

The splint is changed to a cast for a total of 8 weeks of immobilization.

When to Refer

All forearm injuries except for the isolated ulna shaft fracture should be referred within 1 week for possible operative treatment.

Complications

In evaluating patients with forearm fractures, one should be cognizant of compartment syndrome. This is increased pressure within the nonexpandable volar forearm compartment. It is characterized by the five Ps: pain, paresthesias, pressure, pallor, and pulselessness. The earliest and most reliable symptom is pain out of proportion to the injury. The earliest sign is hypoesthesia to light touch in the median nerve distribution (volar thumb). Another

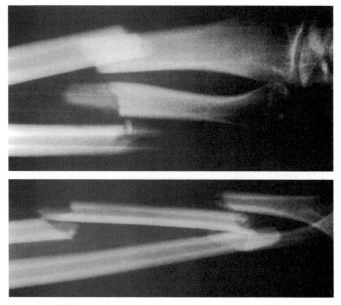

Figure 1 Displaced fractures of both bones of the forearm in a 34-year-old woman as a result of a motor vehicle accident. The radial fracture was segmental.

early sign is pain with passive thumb extension. A compartment syndrome is a surgical emergency requiring fasciotomy and, once suspected, should be emergently referred. Also, immediately remove the cast and Webril.

DISTAL RADIUS FRACTURES

Mechanism of Injury

This injury is very common in the elderly and osteoporotic populations. Most often, one falls on an outstretched hand.

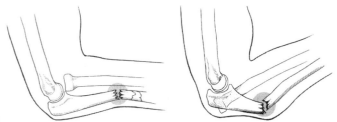

A   B

Figure 2 Bado's classification of Monteggia fractures. **A:** Type I. An anterior dislocation of the radial head with associated anteriorly angulated fracture of the ulna shaft. **B:** Type II. Posterior dislocation of the head with a posteriorly angulated fracture of the ulna. (*continues*)

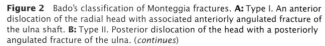

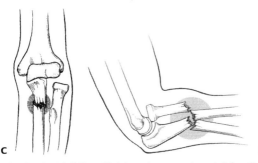

Figure 2 *Continued.* **C:** Type III. A lateral or anterolateral dislocation of the radial head with a fracture of the ulnar metaphysis. **D:** Type IV. Anterior dislocation of the radial head with a fracture of the radius and ulna. (From Bado JL. The Monteggia lesion. *Clin Orthop* 1967;50:70–86, with permission.)

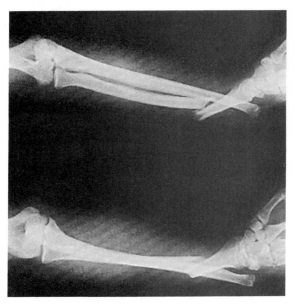

Figure 3 Preoperative anteroposterior and lateral radiographs of a 25-year-old man with a closed Galeazzi fracture. (From Chapman MW, Gordon EJ, Zissimos AG. Compression-plate fixation of acute fractures of the diaphyses of the radius and ulna. *J Bone Joint Surg* 1989;71A:159–169, with permission.)

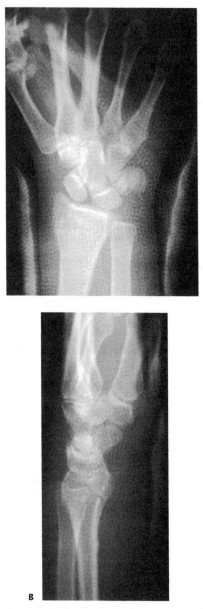

Figure 4 A, B: An extraarticular distal radius fracture managed by cast immobilization. (*continues*)

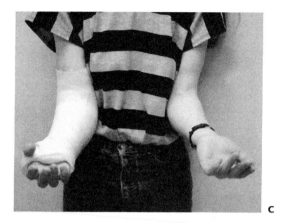

C

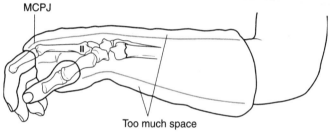

A.1 Poor placement, poor fit

D

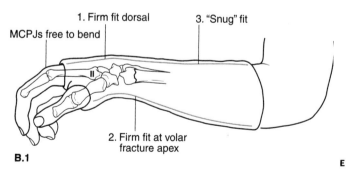

B.1

E

Figure 4 *Continued*. The application of the cast in full supination is seen **(C)**. **D:** A cast applied to the forearm is too distal and can block metacarpophalangeal joint (MCPJ) motion. Care must be taken in cast application to allow for full flexion of all the MCPJs. **E:** An ideal cast is particularly shortened on the palmar aspect so as to allow full finger flexion while offering three-point fracture support. (*continues*)

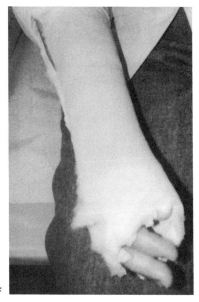

F

Figure 4 *Continued.* **F:** A patient's splint was applied so far distal as to completely block normal thumb function as well as prevent any meaningful finger flexion.

Diagnosis

Pain, swelling, and deformity to the wrist may be evident.

Radiology

Plain anteroposterior and lateral forearm radiographs are satisfactory. These fractures occur through the diaphyseal region of the distal radius. The distal fragment may have displacement and angulation volar or dorsal.

Initial Treatment

Nondisplaced distal radius fractures should be placed in a short-arm cast. Note the importance of stopping the volar distal margin of the cast at the proximal palmar crease. The volar cast margin must be angled at 45 degrees, just like the palmar crease, to allow metacarpophalangeal flexion of the small finger (Fig. 4). Displaced fractures should be reduced in fingertraps with 15 lb of countertraction via stockinette draped over the humerus for 15 minutes (Fig. 5). This allows the fracture to distract and reduce itself. During traction, the proximal and distal fragments are firmly grasped between the index and thumb. The distal fragment is pushed to the edge of the proximal fragment to allow correction of the deformity (Fig. 6). While in traction, a short-arm cast is placed, and a postreduction x-ray is obtained. If reduction is acceptable, the traction is removed after the short-arm cast is hard. Then the cast is extended to a long-arm cast with the elbow in 90-degree flexion (Fig. 7).

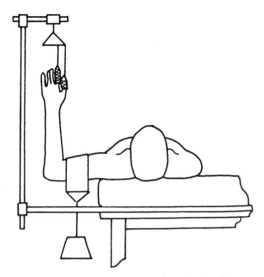

Figure 5 Fingertrap suspension of distal radius fracture.

Definitive Treatment

At 2 weeks, the long-arm cast may be switched to a short-arm cast for another 4 weeks to allow callus formation. Throughout treatment, finger range of motion and strengthening are done.

When to Refer

Patients should be referred when the fracture position before or after reduction is not acceptable. Acceptable reduction requires, on the lateral view, 0 to 15 degrees of volar tilt of the distal radial articular surface. The anteroposterior view must show the radius to be no shorter than the ulna to be acceptable (Fig. 8).

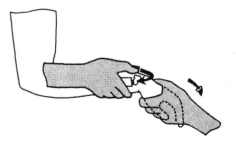

Figure 6 Colles' fracture reduction technique, with manipulation into final reduction.

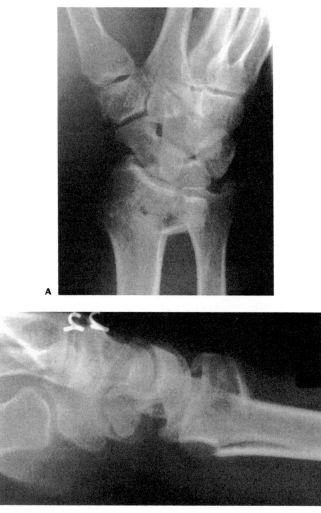

Figure 7 A, B: The inherent instability in shortening of this Colles' fracture is due to the crush of bone that occurred at the time of injury. (*continues*)

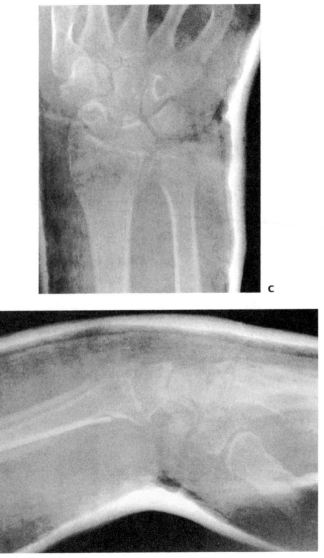

Figure 7 *Continued.* **C, D:** After reduction, the three-point fixation achieved in the cast helps maintain position and length.

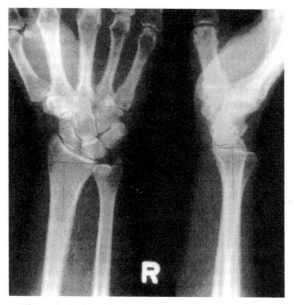

Figure 8 Radiographic parameters of reduction adequacy.

Complications

One should be aware that reductions may be lost during the first 3 weeks of weekly radiographic follow-up. Referral to an orthopedist should be urgent when a loss of reduction is encountered in the first 3 weeks of healing.

Chapter 17

FRACTURES OF THE WRIST AND HAND

Garrick A. Cox and Robert L. Kalb

FRACTURES OF THE CARPAL BONES

Fractures of the radius are often seen in combination with other fractures and dislocations. The scaphoid is the most commonly fractured carpal bone, followed by the triquetrum.

Scaphoid

The scaphoid is the most commonly fractured carpal bone (Fig. 1). The scaphoid receives its blood supply in a distal-to-proximal direction. Therefore, a proximal pole scaphoid fracture has a higher chance of nonunion.

Mechanism of Injury

During wrist hyperextension, the dorsal rim of the radius is driven into the scaphoid. Any displaced fracture of the scaphoid needs surgery.

Diagnosis

Note pain on palpation of the anatomic snuff box.

Radiology

Four views are necessary: anteroposterior with the wrist deviated ulnarward, anteroposterior in radial deviation, oblique, and lateral. Special scaphoid views can be obtained and magnified.

Initial Treatment

If nondisplaced, a thumb spica cast is applied, and the wrist is elevated. If clinical examination suggests a scaphoid fracture (pain in the anatomic snuff box), but no fracture line is seen on x-ray, a thumb spica cast is applied for 2 weeks. At that time, the cast is removed, and repeat scaphoid x-rays are taken. If repeat x-rays are still negative, but clinical tenderness is still present, continue the thumb spica and check again in 3 weeks.

Definitive Treatment

Nondisplaced scaphoid fractures require a long-arm thumb spica cast for 1 month followed by a short-arm thumb spica cast until healing is complete in 2 to 6 months. A computed tomography scan is helpful in determining whether union has occurred. Smokers heal more slowly and have a higher chance of nonunion. All patients with fractures should stop smoking. Any displaced fracture needs surgery.

When to Refer

All displaced fractures should be referred.

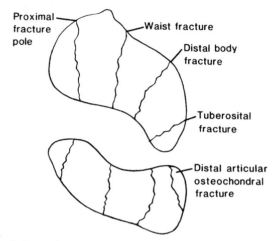

Figure 1   Types of scaphoid fractures. The scaphoid is susceptible to fractures at any level. Approximately 65% occur at the waist, 15% through the proximal pole, 10% through the distal body, 8% through the tuberosity, and 2% in the distal articular surface.

Complications

The most common complications of a scaphoid fracture are nonunion, avascular necrosis, and arthritis. Nonunion and avascular necrosis require surgery. Arthritis is managed with splinting, nonsteroidal antiinflammatory drugs, injection, and activity modification. If these measures fail, surgery can be done.

Fractures of the Other Carpal Bones

Lunate, capitate, triquetrum, and pisiform fractures are all much less common than scaphoid fractures. A fracture should be definitively ruled out before a diagnosis of strain, sprain, or contusion is made. These fractures are most often chip or avulsion fractures and can be treated conservatively with a short-arm cast for comfort and protection for 1 month until symptoms resolve. Any fracture with displacement of the articular surface should be referred.

METACARPAL FRACTURES

Metacarpal fractures involve the base, shaft, neck, or head of the metacarpal. It is important to note additional factors such as open wounds, dislocations, and whether more than one metacarpal is fractured.

Diagnosis

Pain and often deformity are localized to the area of injury. Always confirm rotational alignment of all digits. Digital overlap may occur in metacarpal fractures if they are not immobilized with the metacarpophalangeal joints flexed 90 degrees.

Radiology

Anteroposterior, lateral, and oblique views of the hand are obtained.

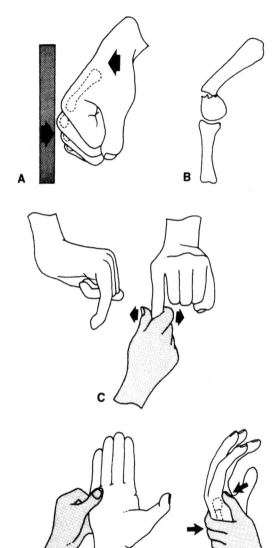

Figure 2 Boxer fracture of the fifth metacarpal and reduction technique.
A: Mechanism of injury. **B:** Dorsal angulation. **C:** Disimpaction of fragments.
D: Reduction maneuver.

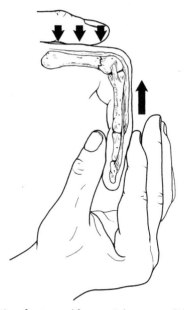

Figure 3 Reduction of metacarpal fractures is best accomplished by using the straight digit to exert a dorsally directed force through the metacarpophalangeal joint while viewing the digit as a lever arm that indicates correct rotational alignment of the metacarpal fracture.

Reasons for Operative Intervention

Operative intervention should take place in the following situations:
- Boxer fractures (fifth metacarpal neck fractures) with greater than 40 degrees of persistent angulation after reduction
- Angulation of metacarpal shaft fractures greater than 10 degrees
- Intraarticular displaced fractures involving the thumb joints
- Carpal-metacarpal dislocations
- Any malrotation that cannot be corrected

Treatment of Nondisplaced Fractures

Even if nondisplaced fractures are intraarticular, they should be treated with a gutter splint. Fractures of the thumb metacarpal should be treated with a spica cast. An index metacarpal fracture can be treated with a radial gutter splint with a hole cut out for the thumb to allow function. Fractures of the middle, ring, and small metacarpal should be treated with an ulnar gutter splint for 1 month.

Boxer Fractures

Boxer fractures occur at the small-finger metacarpal neck (Fig. 2). Angulation greater than 40 degrees should be reduced (Fig. 3). An ulnar gutter splint is used for 3 weeks followed by range of motion twice a day.

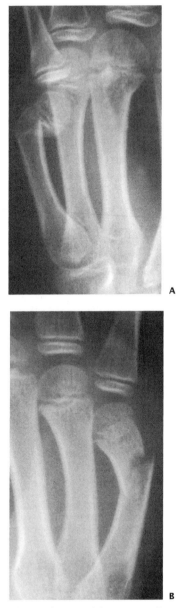

Figure 4 **A:** A true boxer's fracture of the metacarpal neck of the fifth ray. **B:** This fracture occurs more in the diaphysis and should not be considered a boxer's fracture.

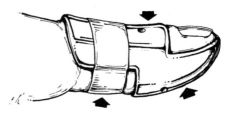

Figure 5   Stack splint.

Associated Injuries of Metacarpal Fractures

Any wound over the metacarpal head warrants clinical suspicion of a "fight bite" or punch to the mouth. These injuries have a high infection rate and often require surgical irrigation and débridement (Fig. 4).

Complications

Complications of metacarpal fractures include malunion, nonunion, and tendon adhesions. Malunions and nonunions need to be corrected operatively. Adhesions are managed initially with intensive physical therapy. If this fails, surgical release may be necessary.

FINGERS

All nondisplaced fractures can be buddy taped for 1 month. Refer all intraarticular displaced fractures. Dorsal extensor tendon avulsions at the distal interphalangeal joint (mallet finger) with or without bone avulsion are treated with a stack splint (Fig. 5) for 8 weeks. If the splint is removed, the finger tip must be held in full extension until the splint is replaced.

Chapter 18

PEDIATRIC FRACTURES

Garrick A. Cox and Robert L. Kalb

HOW TO RECOGNIZE FRACTURES

The diagnosis of a fracture in a child may be difficult. Often, radiographs do not show a fracture, and the diagnosis is made clinically by point tenderness over the growth plate. If point tenderness is located over a growth plate, a fracture is present. The purpose of doing an x-ray is to determine if the fracture is displaced or not.

The indication for obtaining an x-ray in an adult or a child is point tenderness over the bone, deformity, and inability to bear weight on the injured extremity. If a patient does not have point tenderness over the bone at the site of injury and there is no pain associated with weight bearing, a radiograph is not required.

In children, ligaments are stronger than the growth plate cartilage (physis or epiphysis). The growth plate should be thought of as the weakest link, designed to fail first. The physis will crack before a ligament tear can occur in children. For this reason, one should not make a diagnosis of a sprain in a child.

BONE

Children's bones are elastic, similar to a plastic fly-swatter handle. Their bones can be deformed and bow without cracking the cortex. This "plastic" deformation occurs in the radial and ulnar shafts during forearm injuries. This is commonly referred to as a *both-bone forearm bow fracture.* It is seen in children younger than 3 years of age, when the bones are the most malleable. Pediatric bones can also bow enough to crack only one cortex. This is referred to as a *green-stick fracture.* (If you try to break a green branch off a tree, it may only break on one side, hence the term *green-stick.*)

If you are ever in doubt about the normal alignment of the forearm, remember that the ulna is always straight, and there is a small 10- to 20-degree dorsal bow present normally in the radius. You can also determine normal alignment by obtaining a comparison radiograph of the normal uninjured side. Always make sure that the views are taken with the arms in the same position of rotation, flexion, and extension for accurate comparison. Comparison views are important when treating any elbow injury because of the numerous centers of ossification in the elbow that develop through age 15 years.

SALTER-HARRIS CLASSIFICATION

The Salter-Harris classification system (Fig. 1) is based on fracture patterns to the growth plate. The end of a long bone is the *epiphysis.* The growth plate is the *epiphyseal plate* (physis). The flare of the bone below the physis is the *metaphysis.* The shaft of the bone is the *diaphysis.*

Salter-Harris Type I

Salter-Harris type I is a fracture through the physis; the x-ray is normal. This fracture type is diagnosed by point tenderness over the growth plate. These fractures are common in infants and young children. Treatment is a cast.

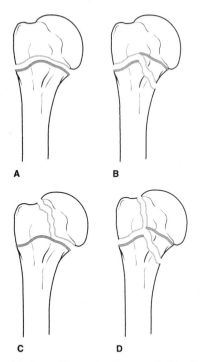

Figure 1   Physeal fractures of the proximal humerus. **A:** Salter-Harris I. **B:** Salter-Harris II. **C:** Salter-Harris III. **D:** Salter-Harris IV.

Salter-Harris Type II

The Salter-Harris type II fracture pattern (Fig. 2) involves a fracture line that crosses the growth plate and exits the metaphysis. These fractures are more common in older children. The prognosis for growth disturbance is highest when it involves the distal femoral growth plate. These fractures are displaced and should be referred. An orthopedic referral for operative reduction under general anesthesia is warranted.

Salter-Harris Type III

The Salter-Harris type III fracture (Fig. 3) involves the epiphysis and the epiphyseal plate. This is an intraarticular fracture, and if there is any displacement, operative intervention is necessary. These are most commonly seen in the distal tibia and have a higher association with growth arrest than the previous two fracture types. Anatomic reduction is the goal.

Salter-Harris Type IV

As in Salter-Harris type III fractures, Salter-Harris type IV injuries are intraarticular and need to be anatomically aligned. If the fracture appears nondisplaced but there is question of displacement, an orthopedist should be consulted to view the film.

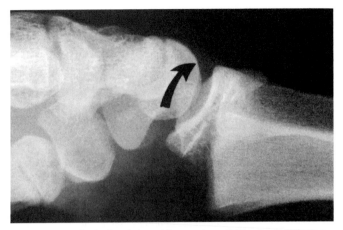

Figure 2   Dorsally displaced physeal fracture (type A). The distal epiphysis with a small metaphyseal fragment is displaced dorsally (*arrow*) in relation to the proximal metaphyseal fragment.

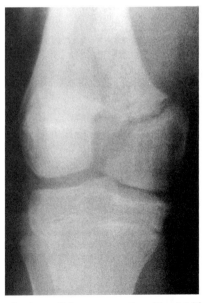

Figure 3   Salter-Harris type III fracture separation of the distal femur. Note the vertical fracture line extending from the growth plate distally into the intercondylar notch with displacement.

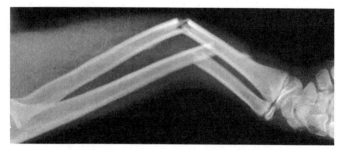

Figure 4   Apex volar angulation of 45 degrees.

ABUSE

Any suspicious history indicating child abuse should be investigated by taking long-bone radiographs of the upper and lower extremities. These films should be inspected for signs of fractures in various bones at different stages of healing. A corner fracture is commonly associated with child abuse. This fracture is located at the corner of the metaphysis of long bones. These are most often seen around the distal femur and proximal tibia. Other fractures that are linked with abuse are humerus, femur, and rib fractures.

REFERRING CHILDREN WITH FRACTURES

As with adult bone injuries, children with any open fractures should be referred to an orthopedist. An open fracture may be associated with only a small puncture wound in the skin. This puncture wound may be located several inches from the fracture itself due to the forces of deformation at the time of injury. Children with fractures involving the spine or knee should also be referred because of the high risk of neurologic injury and growth plate arrest. You should always obtain comparison views for any fracture about the elbow. Because the elbow has delayed centers of ossification, refer patients to an orthopedist to review the films. Children who have any fractures with intraarticular displacement should be referred.

FRACTURES OF THE RADIAL AND ULNAR SHAFT, TIBIA, AND FIBULA

Fractures of the radial and ulnar shaft (Fig. 4) or tibia (Fig. 5) should always be referred if there is displacement greater than 50% or angulation greater than 10 degrees. Treatment for these fractures includes a long-arm or long-leg cast. The cast should remain in place 4 to 8 weeks depending on the child's age.

CLAVICLE FRACTURES

Children with clavicle fractures do not require reduction. Referral should be considered for displaced distal clavicle fractures near the acromioclavicular joint or proximal fractures near the sternum, or if there is tenting of the skin from the fractured fragments. Most fractures, however, occur in the mid-third of the clavicle and are usually treated with a simple sling or a figure-of-eight

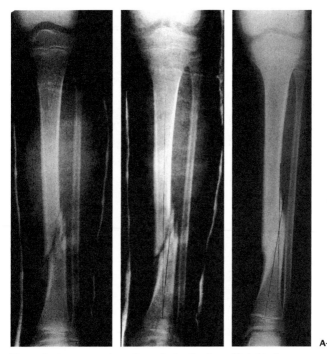

A–C

Figure 5 Anteroposterior radiograph of a distal one-third tibia fracture without a concomitant fibula fracture in a 10-year-old child. **A:** The alignment in the coronal plane is acceptable (note that the proximal and distal tibial growth plates are parallel). **B:** A varus angulation developed within the first 2 weeks after injury. **C:** At radiographic union, a 10-degree varus angulation is present and acceptable because, with bone growth, it will straighten.

strap. For older children, a sling may be more comfortable than a figure-of-eight strap.

FRACTURES OF THE SHOULDER

Fractures of the shoulder most commonly involve the surgical neck of the humerus. Reduction or manipulation of this fracture is usually not necessary as long as there is at least 50% bone-on-bone contact and fewer than 45 degrees of angulation. Treatment includes a coaptation splint and sling for 3 weeks until tenderness resolves on palpation.

Humeral shaft fractures (Fig. 6) heal well with angulation as high as 25 degrees on anteroposterior and lateral views. Just as for adults, the fracture should be immobilized initially in a coaptation splint and then converted to a humeral fracture brace (Fig. 7). These fractures usually take 6 weeks to heal. There is an association with radial nerve palsy and humeral shaft fractures. Radial nerve function can be tested by asking the patient to extend the thumb, fingers, and the wrist. Radial sensation is tested in the dorsal first web space.

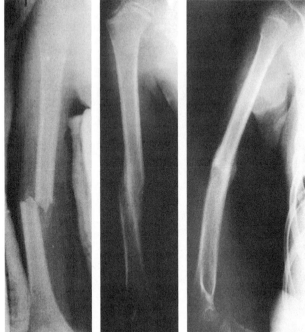

A–C

Figure 6   A: Humerus fracture allowed to heal in slight varus and bayonet application. **B, C:** The ultimate result, with essentially normal alignment.

DISTAL HUMERUS
SUPRACONDYLAR FRACTURES

The distal humerus ordinarily has a tilt in an anterior direction of 30 degrees. On a lateral radiograph, draw a line down the anterior humeral cortex. This line should bisect the capitellum at the level of the elbow. Supracondylar fractures (Fig. 8) as well as radial head/neck fractures (Fig. 9) are sometimes not obvious on radiographs. A posterior fat pad (sail sign) is a dark shadow behind the distal humerus. It is secondary to hemarthrosis from the fracture. This causes the fat pad, hiding in the posterior elbow trochlea, to float out and become visible on x-ray. An anterior fat pad is normal and does not signify a fracture. If there is no tenderness over the distal humerus, make sure you palpate the radial head. For fractures of the radial head and neck, the acceptable range of angulation is 30 degrees.

BUCKLE FRACTURES OF THE DISTAL RADIUS

Buckle fractures of the distal radius are the most common fracture (Fig. 10) in pediatrics. They are caused by a fall onto an outstretched hand, causing the distal radius to "buckle." These fractures are stable but have the potential for displacement. They are treated in a short-arm cast for 4 weeks.

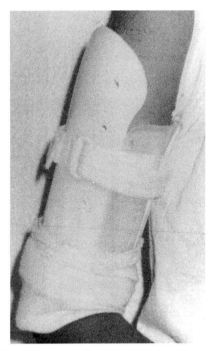

Figure 7 Light, plastic, functional braces are useful to maintain alignment and allow early restoration of motion, particularly in older children and adolescents.

FRACTURES OF THE CARPAL BONES

Fractures of the carpal bones are uncommon in children. A fall onto an outstretched arm is the most typical mechanism. The scaphoid (Fig. 11) is the most common carpal bone fractured. It is diagnosed clinically by tenderness in the anatomic snuff box. Snuff box tenderness requires a thumb spica cast for a minimum of 2 weeks and a repeat scaphoid view. Often, this second x-ray at 2 weeks shows the fracture line. These fractures require 6 weeks of immobilization in a short-arm cast

METACARPAL AND PHALANGEAL FRACTURES

Metacarpal and phalangeal fractures that are nondisplaced can often be treated with an ulnar gutter splint. The position of immobilization is metacarpal flexion of 90 degrees and distal interphalangeal and proximal interphalangeal straight.

FRACTURES OF THE PELVIS
AND FEMORAL SHAFT

Fractures of the pelvis are uncommon and are usually associated with high-velocity trauma. Patients with these fractures should be referred to a trauma center to rule out other associated injuries.

Fractures of the femur should be immediately referred.

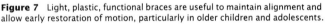

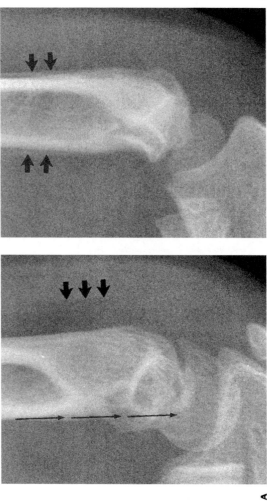

Figure 8 Supracondylar fractures. **A:** Where the anterior humeral line (*thin arrows*) normally crosses through the ossification center of the capitellum. There is also posterior displacement of the olecranon fat pad (*large arrows*). **B:** Three weeks postinjury, there is evidence of new periosteal bone formation from both the anterior and posterior cortices (*arrows*). Because a definite fracture line was not seen in the original radiographs, this new bone formation confirms the original suspicion of a fracture. (*continues*)

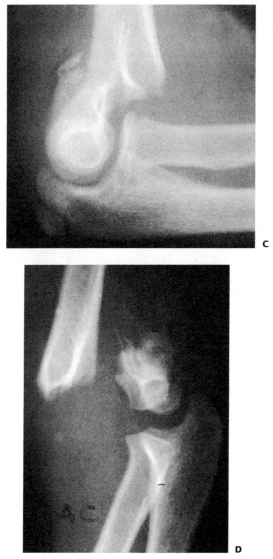

Figure 8 *Continued.* **C:** Type II. Lateral view of a displaced supracondylar fracture with the posterior cortex intact. There are both rotation and angulation of the distal fragment. **D:** Type III. Totally displaced fracture. There is no contact between the fragments. **C** and **D** require referral for reduction.

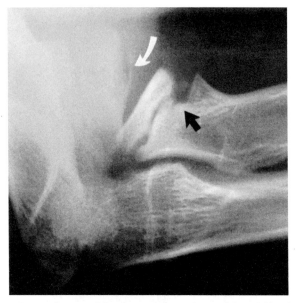

Figure 9 Angular stress deformity: anterior angulation of the radial head and neck in a 12-year-old pitcher. There is evidence of some disruption of the normal growth of the anterior portion of the physis (*black arrow*). The capitellum also demonstrates radiographic signs of osteochondritis dissecans (*white arrow*). (Courtesy of Kenneth P. Butters, M.D.)

PATELLAR FRACTURES

Patellar fractures are usually the result of a direct blow. They are usually nondisplaced and treated with a knee immobilizer. This remains in place for 4 weeks, and then range of motion exercises are begun. There is a patellar variant that is often confused with a fractured patella (bipartite patella). This is an unfused portion of the patella in the upper lateral quadrant. It is often bilateral. It is not point tender to touch as it would be if it were a fracture.

TIBIAL SPINE FRACTURES IN THE KNEE

Intraarticular avulsion fractures (Fig. 12) of the intercondylar eminence indicate the anterior cruciate ligament has been avulsed. If there is displacement, the patient should be referred.

FRACTURES OF THE TIBIA, FIBULA, AND ANKLE

Proximal tibia fractures are treated in the same manner as those of the distal femur and are diagnosed by point tenderness over the growth plate. Nondisplaced tibial shaft fractures can be treated in a long-leg cast without reduction, provided that there is no greater than 5 degrees of angulation on the anteroposterior view and 10 degrees on the lateral view. Fractures with greater angulation require reduction.

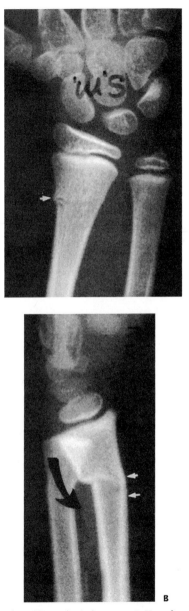

Figure 10   Metaphyseal biomechanical patterns. **A:** Torus fracture. Simple bulging of the thin cortex (*arrow*). **B:** Compression green-stick fracture. Angulation of the dorsal cortex (*large curved arrow*). The volar cortex is intact but slightly plastically deformed (*small white arrows*).

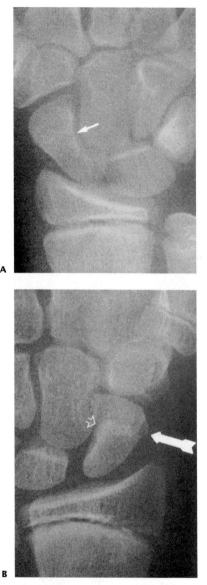

Figure 11   A: A barely detectable fracture line is located in the mid-waist of the scaphoid (*arrow*). **B:** In contrast, this mid-waist scaphoid fracture has occurred at the junction of the middle and distal thirds. Articulation between the scaphoid and capitate has been rendered incongruous by displacement of the distal pole (*open arrow*). There is mild comminution in the radial aspect (*closed arrow*).

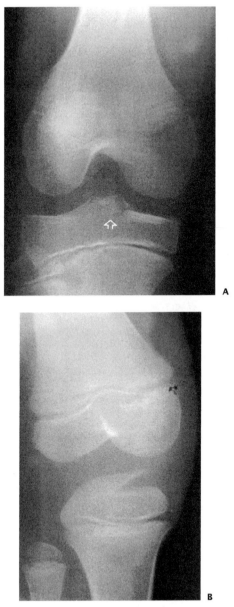

Figure 12 Stages of displacement of tibial spine fractures. **A:** Type I fracture, minimal displacement (*open arrow*). **B:** Type II fracture, posterior hinge intact. (*continues*)

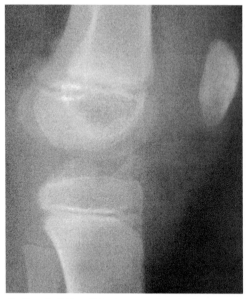

C

Figure 12 *Continued.* **C:** Type III fracture, complete displacement and proximal migration.

Nondisplaced fibular fractures heal well with a short-leg walking cast for 6 weeks. All displaced fractures should be referred.

FRACTURES OF THE FOOT

Fractures of the talus are often associated with avascular necrosis. If nondisplaced, they can be treated in a non–weight-bearing short-leg cast for a minimum of 12 weeks. If there is any displacement, they are referred. Fractures of the tarsal navicular and cuneiform bones can be treated with a short-leg walking cast, provided there is no displacement.

Fractures of the metatarsals are treated in the same manner as in adults. Base of the fifth metatarsal avulsion fractures (peroneus brevis avulsion) can be treated with a wooden sole fracture shoe.

A Jones fracture is through the junction of the metaphysis and diaphysis of the proximal fifth metatarsal. This fracture can go on to nonunion and should be treated in a non–weight-bearing short-leg cast for a minimum of 6 weeks and then with full weight bearing for 6 more weeks in the cast.

Chapter 19

CASTING

Richard B. Birrer

Physicians who manage fractures need to know how to apply a cast and splint. Plaster does not produce allergies. It is inexpensive in comparison with fiberglass and is most adaptable to the part being splinted. It is applied with or without gloves. Its disadvantage is that it is slow to dry and gain full strength. It can be seriously weakened if it becomes wet once it is dry. Plaster is very heavy when wet but becomes lighter when dry. Because it is partially radio-opaque, bone details on radiographs can be obscured.

Fiberglass is light, waterproof, and durable but requires airtight packaging. It must be applied while wearing gloves. It does not splash like plaster and hardens rapidly by exposure to water over a period of 10 minutes. It is three times more expensive than plaster, but because of its strength, fewer rolls are required. Fiberglass is radiolucent and lighter weight.

CAST APPLICATION

Tubular stockinette (Figs. 1 and 2) can be used to cover the skin. Extra layers of Webril should be placed over bony prominences. The appropriate size of plaster roll is then chosen—for the lower extremities, 4-in. and 6-in. widths and 2-in. to 4-in. on upper extremity injuries. For children, choose 2 in. and 4 in. for the lower and 2 in. for the upper extremity, depending on the size of the child. The plaster bandage is then unwound for approximately 10 cm (4 in.), and both the roll and the free end are held under the water for 30 seconds until bubbles cease to rise.

Cold water is used to extend the setting time and warm water to shorten it. The plaster splint is then carefully lifted out of the water and gently squeezed with the bandage drawn through both finger and thumb to wring out the water (Fig. 3). It can then be wrapped around the part to be casted. The wet plaster bandage is always applied distally, proceeding proximally, thus diminishing venous congestion and allowing smoother application of the bandage. A thick layer of Webril 3 cm long should be left to protrude beyond the margins of the plaster. The circles of wet plaster bandage are tucked (Figs. 4 and 5) where a limb circumference enlarges (proximal forearm or calf of the leg). A 50% overlap of width gives a double layer of plaster, and 60% overlap gives a triple layer. At the proximal and distal edge, the Webril is folded back to give a smooth edge with full movement for the fingers and toes (Fig. 6). To fit the limb accurately, the plaster is then smoothed and molded (Fig. 7).

The injured limb should be elevated on folded blankets with the hip and knee each flexed at 90 degrees. The neurovascular status is checked regularly. The patient should return the next day for inspection of the limb and the cast. A set of cast instructions should be given to the patient to identify danger signs. Information about care of the cast and exercises for the leg is included.

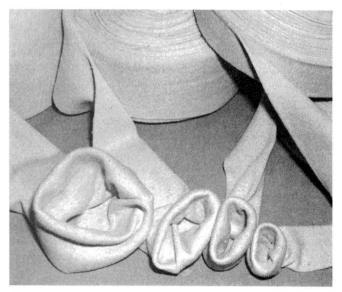

Figure 1 Tubular stockinette is used to line and trim the end of casts, and it has many other uses. It is available in widths from 2 to 12 in.

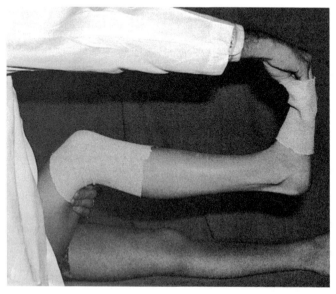

Figure 2 Tubular stockinette used to trim the ends of a short-leg cast.

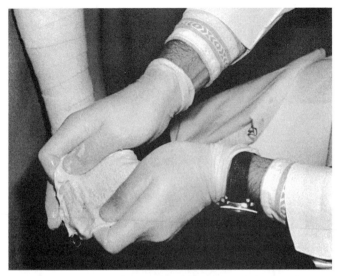

Figure 3 Gently squeeze the water out of the roll by accordioning it from either side. Twisting or manipulating the roll results in excessive loss of plaster.

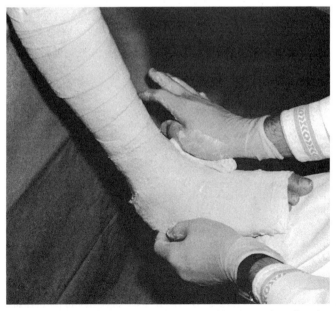

A

Figure 4 **A:** Begin with a 4-in. roll at the metatarsal heads; use this roll on the foot and ankle. Notice that the plaster roll is pushed, not pulled. (*continues*)

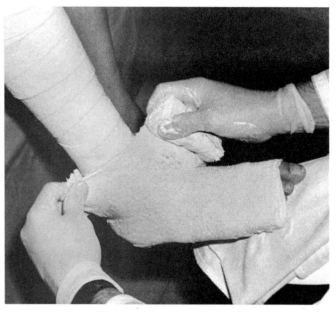

B

Figure 4 *Continued.* **B:** To change the direction of the roll, place the leading edge in the direction you want the roll to go. This maneuver produces a loose corner of plaster, seen here in the surgeon's left hand. Take a tuck with the left hand and smooth it down on the posterior aspect of the leg. For sharp changes of direction, pick up the roll with the right hand, but in general leave the roll on the extremity.

SPLINT APPLICATION

Splints are used under the following circumstances:

- Reinforcement of circular casts to strengthen high-stress areas (e.g., at a joint).
- Initial splinting of soft tissue injuries or fractures, because splints are easily applied and allow more space for swelling of the limb than a cast.

The splint can be fashioned out of circular bandage, which is time consuming, or multiple layers of bandage are available as splints. The required length is pulled out of the box and cut off. To create a splint from a roll, a flat, dry surface is used, on which the material is unrolled and doubled backward and forward on itself to form a splint of the required length and thickness. Tubular stockinette and Webril padding to protect the skin and skeletal prominences are first applied. The splinting material is laid on the padding, leaving the distal and proximal 4 cm free of splint material. These soft padded ends are turned back later to form a smooth padded edge. The splint is held in place by a wet plaster or fiberglass roll, which is applied with even tension working distally to proximally, because this direction helps to diminish the swelling of the extremity. The cast is then completed with proximal and distal edges turned back and smoothly held in place by the exterior roll (Figs. 4, 5, 6, 8, 9, 10, 11, 12, 13, 14, and 15).

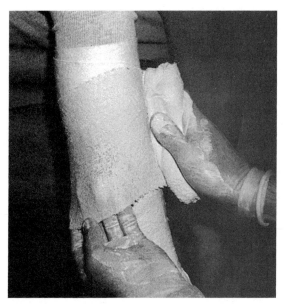

Figure 5 On the midportion of the limb, take tucks by slipping the hand under the near edge of the plaster and sliding it until it is transverse to the long axis of the limb. Smooth out the tuck posteriorly and continue rolling.

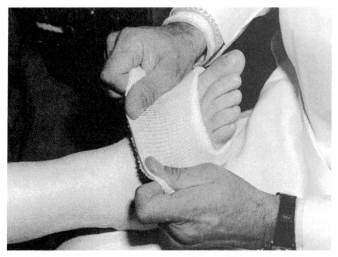

Figure 6 When tubular stockinette is used, trim the edge of the cast just distal to the metatarsal heads, turn back a layer of Webril to pad the end of the cast, and turn back the tubular stockinette, securing it in place with a few wraps of circumferential plaster.

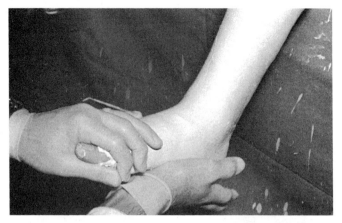

Figure 7 Once all the plaster has been applied and rubbed in, begin molding at the foot. Restore the longitudinal and transverse arches of the foot.

REMOVAL OF CAST OR SPLINT

A splint can be easily removed by using a pair of scissors to cut the padding and Ace wrap. Casts are more difficult to remove as there is a possibility of damaging the patient's skin. It is an advantage to have an assistant hold the cast steady to prevent movement by the patient.

The removal of a cast is done with an oscillating saw, of which there are several models. Because of the vibration and noise, patients, particularly children, are afraid of being cut by the saw. The saw does not damage skin provided that it is not pulled along the skin surface. If the skin is very thin and

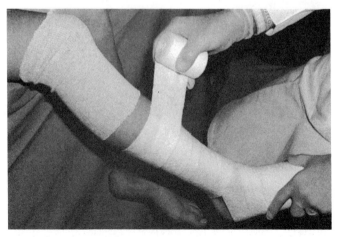

Figure 8 Application of Webril. Hold the Webril off the extremity and apply it with tension to achieve a smooth wrap two to four layers thick.

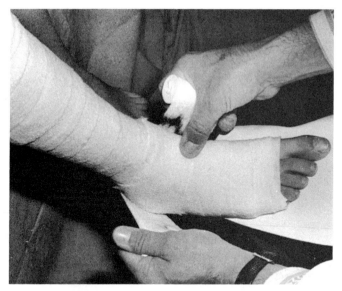

Figure 9 Pad the heel with separate strips of Webril.

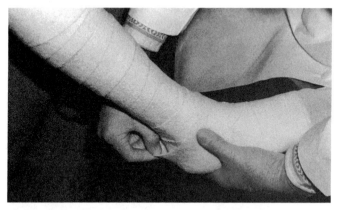

Figure 10 When applying Webril, loose edges can be smoothed by simply pulling them away.

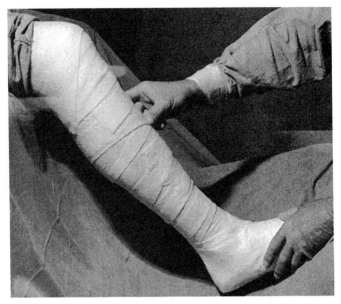

Figure 11   The Webril padding has been completed.

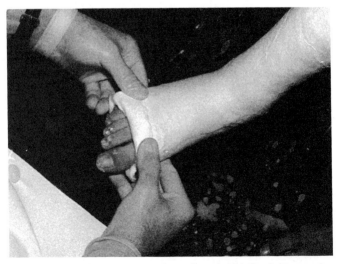

Figure 12   If tubular stockinette is not used, cut the Webril and plaster on the lateral and medial aspects and turn them back to produce a soft cuff, which is then secured with a few turns of fresh plaster.

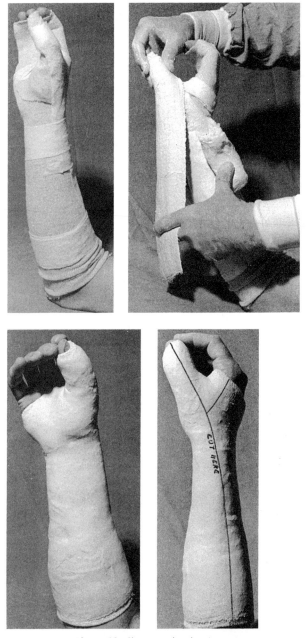

Figure 13 Short-arm thumb spica cast.

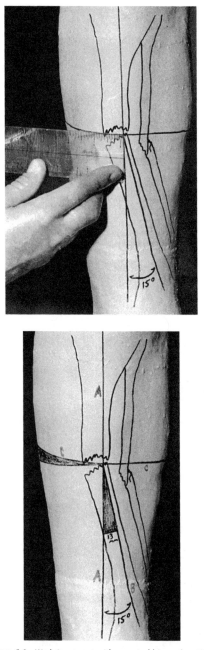

Figure 14 Wedging a cast with a central hinge. (*continues*)

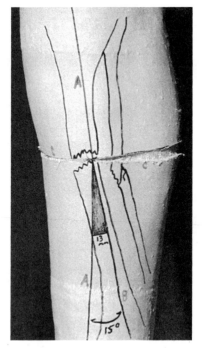

Figure 14 *Continued.*

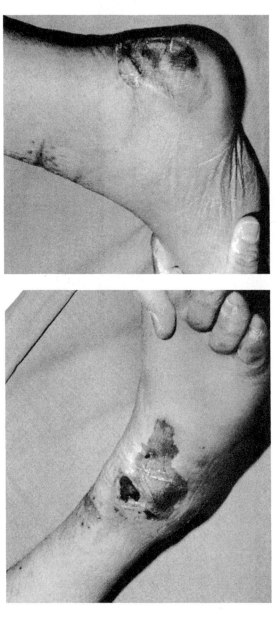

Figure 15 These pressure sores over the instep and heel of the foot were caused by a long-leg cast applied to a patient with a fracture of the proximal tibia who was multiply injured and unconscious for 3 days. Although the initial cast was probably applied in an appropriate manner, subsequent swelling in the cast, about which the patient could not complain, led to these pressure ulcers. These full-thickness ulcers resulted in exposure of the Achilles tendon and calcaneus and full exposure of the extensor tendons of the ankle; major plastic reconstructive surgery was required. These problems could have been avoided by univalving the cast and spreading it widely initially, or by using splints with frequent inspection of the skin.

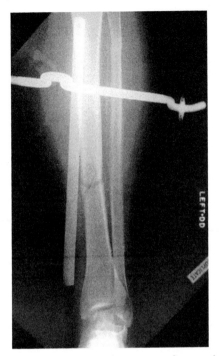

Figure 16 In stable fractures such as this transverse fracture, shortening is rarely a problem, but care must be taken to avoid angulation and malrotation.

fragile, as in elderly patients or those with rheumatoid arthritis, there is increased risk for skin damage. Serious damage can be caused to the skin of an unconscious patient, especially if the blade is hot.

A line of cut is chosen that avoids any skeletal prominences. The blade is carefully introduced between the bandage and skin. Small, regular cuts are then made without digging the blade into the patient's skin. The oscillating cast saw should be held so that there is no danger of the blade coming into contact with the skin. Only the plaster is cut. Padding oscillates with the blade and is not cut. The blade can become hot and should be allowed to cool. Dull blades become hot sooner. Bivalving a cast makes its removal easy. When using the saw, the blade must always be moved away from the electrical cord to avoid damage. The two halves of the cast can be separated by using the cast spreader. On removing a cast, care must be taken not to lever on the mobile fracture site or a stiff joint. The back half of a cast can be used for transferring the patient for x-ray and for a removable splint to allow intermittent joint movement. Skin lotion can be used to soften the skin on cast removal because normal desquamation has been prevented by the cast. The skin softens, and the dry top layer flakes off after several washings (Fig. 16).

BIBLIOGRAPHY

Bucholz RW, Heckman, eds. *Rockwood and Green's fractures in adults*, 5th ed. Philadelphia: Lippincott Williams & Wilkins, 2002.

Canale ST. *Campbell's operative orthopaedics*, 10th ed. Vol 3. Philadelphia: Mosby, 2003.

Chapman MW, ed. *Chapman's orthopaedic surgery*, 3rd ed. Vols 1–4. Philadelphia: Lippincott Williams & Wilkins, 2001.

Eiff MP. Management of clavicle fractures. *Am Fam Physician* 1997;55(1):121–128.

England SP, Sundberg S. Management of common pediatric fractures. *Pediatr Clin North Am* 1996;44(1):991–1012.

Hatch RL, Hacking S. Evaluation and management of toe fractures. *Am Fam Physician* 2003;68(12):2413–2418.

Moehring H, Greenspan A. *Fractures: diagnosis and treatment*, 4th ed. Philadelphia: McGraw-Hill, 2000.

Perron AD, Brady WJ, Keats TA. Management of common stress fractures. When to apply conservative therapy, when to take an aggressive approach. *Postgrad Med* 2002;111(2):95–96, 99–100, 105–106.

Perry C, Elstrom J. *Handbook of fractures*, 2nd ed. Philadelphia: McGraw-Hill, 2000.

Sanderlin BW, Raspa RF. Common stress fractures. *Am Fam Physician* 2003;68(8):1527–1532.

Solomon L, Nayagam D, Warwick D. *Apley's system of orthopaedics and fractures*, 8th ed. London: Butterworth-Heinemann, 2001.

Strayer SM, Reece SG, Petrizzi MJ. Fractures of the proximal fifth metatarsal. *Am Fam Physician* 1999;59(9):2516–2522.

Townsend DJ, Bassett GS. Common elbow fractures in children. *Am Fam Physician* 1996;53(6):2031–2041.

Note: Page numbers followed by *f* indicate figures; those followed by *t* indicate tables.

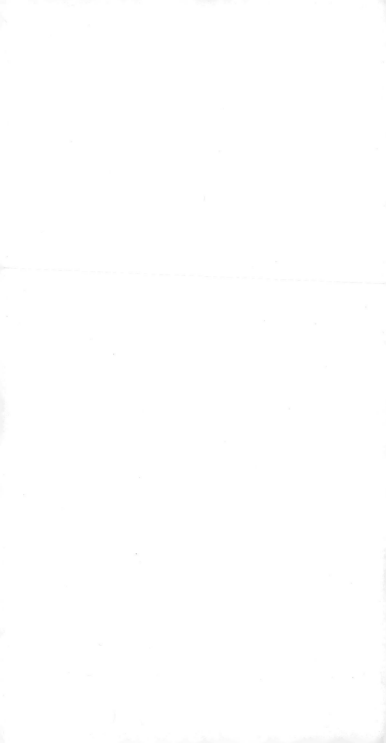